Preface and Acknowledgements

This book is basically the result of nine years of teaching materials to Chinese herbal medicine students. This book is dedicated to the many good, sincere students we have taught in our herbology class over the years. Some of the graduates have also been acupuncturists and doctors in Florida or other states in the US. Some of the graduates have also been practicing very successfully in the clinic. We are very grateful to them for their patience and tolerance as it progressed from crude notes to its present form. The material owes its existence to many conversations and collaborations with our students and many more hours of reading and reviewing this book. Here, we would like to express our special thanks to Cathy Claussell and Arianne Inchausti-lyon, two of our students who contributed to the proofreading of the current edition.

There are a lot of Chinese herbal books available in the market, however, most of them are fit to be as reference books instead of text books for TCM school students. As we know, most TCM students in the US are part-time and they need to concentrate on the most useful and succinct information in order to grasp the knowledge more efficiently. For this reason, we work together and co-edit this book.

Most of the key points that are bold printed are important in this book. Practice questions attached behind every section or chapter will help students digest the relating contents. We hope this book can also contribute to students for preparing for License Examination in the future.

After being published, we hope this book can help more people study Traditional Chinese Medicine. We are thankful for any strong reactions, both positive and negative, from you!

Yu Qi

Dongcheng Li

August, 2013

Copyright

Cover design by Yu Qi and Dongcheng Li
Book design by Yu Qi and Dongcheng Li
Edit by Yu Qi and Dongcheng Li
Cover page picture by Yu Qi and Dongcheng Li

Printed in the United States of America
Fifth Printing: August, 2013
ISBN-13: 978-1456481469
ISBN-10: 1456481460

Contents

Introduction

The Herbal Medicine of Traditional Chinese Medicine (TCM) is the study of sources, collections, properties, actions, indications, contraindications and clinical applications of Chinese natural herbal medicine based on basic theories of Traditional Chinese Medicine. It is one of the most important parts of Traditional Chinese Medicine. In China, 80% of TCM doctors work with herbal medicine, only 20% of them work with acupuncture.

According to a recent survey, the total number of Chinese herbal medicines used is 12,807, in which 11,146 are of plant origin, 1,581 are of animal origin and 80 are of mineral origin. Because most Chinese natural medicines are of plant origin, they are called "Chinese herbal medicines" or "herbs".

In Chinese language, Chinese natural medicine is called "Zhong Yao Xue" 中药学, means "Chinese Herbal Medicine." Among them "Zhong" 中 means Chinese, "Yao" 药 means herbal medicine that can treat diseases, and "Xue" 学 means -ology, a study of.

Western medicine came into China only about 100 years ago. From prehistoric times to the early 20th century, Chinese herbs played a leading role in preventing and treating diseases for Chinese people. They saved many lives. This is one of the important reasons that the population of China is the largest in the world.

In China there are about 30 public TCM universities and many TCM departments in western medical and pharmaceutical universities. There is a department of TCM pharmacology in every public TCM university. Graduates form these departments are pharmacists working for pharmaceutical company or pharmacies.

With the use of modern pharmacology techniques, Chinese herbal medicine is more scientific now. It can be divided into a series of branches:

1) Pharmacognosy: The branch of pharmacology that deals with drugs in their crude or natural state.
2) Phytochemistry: The chemistry of plants.
3) Pharmaceutics: The science of preparing and dispensing drugs.
4) Clinical pharmacology.
5) Formulations of TCM.
6) Herbal processing of TCM.

1. Origin and development of Chinese Herbal Medicine

Chinese Herbal Medicine originated in ancient times when people were looking for food.

There is legend that 5000 years ago there was a ruler called Shen Nong (divine husbandman) who taught his people how to cultivate grains as food so as to avoid killing animals. He tasted 70 herbs a day to test their medical value for his people. He is considered to be the father of Chinese agriculture and herbal medicine.

In the Shang Dynasty (16th - 11th century BC) the letter “Yao” (药) appeared, which means herbs that can treat diseases.

In the Zhou Dynasty (11th century BC - 221 BC) the position of doctor was named officially. Wan Wu (万物 means everything in the world) was written. There are 70 herbs were described in it.

In the Qin and Han Dynasty (221 BC - 220) **Divine Husbandman's Classic of Chinese Herbal Medicine (Shin Nong Ben Cao Jing)** was written, which contains details of 365 herbs. It is the earliest and one of the most valuable books of Chinese Herbal Medicine. More than 200 herbs in current herbal text books are from this book.

In the Three Kingdoms Period, Jin Dynasty, Northern and Southern Dynasties (220 - 589) the important books entitled Ben Cao Jin Ji Zhu and Pao Jiu Lun were written.

In the Sui and Tang Dynasty (581 - 907), the book Newly Revised Chinese Herbal Medicine (Xin Xiu Ben Cao) was published.

In the Song dynasty the state owned pharmacies were established, In Song, Liao, Jin, and Yuan Dynasty (960 - 1368), total herbal medicines reached 1700 different kinds.

In the Ming Dynasty (1368 - 1644) **Grand Chinese Herbal Medicine (Ben Cao Gang Mu)** was written in 1590 AC. It contains details of 1892 Chinese herbal medications.

In the time of the Republic of China (1911 - 1949), the Encyclopedia of Chinese Herbal Medicine (Zhong Yao Da Chi Dian) was compiled, which included 4300 items.

During the People’s Republic of China (1949 – present), TCM universities have been established since 1956 and since then, departments of pharmacology of Traditional Chinese Medication were established in TCM universities. Pharmacology universities and Agriculture universities, and many books were published including Chinese Herbal Medicine (Zhong Hua Ben Cao), the 8534 herbal medicine listed.

2. Habitat and collection of Chinese Herbal Medicine

2.1 Habitat of Chinese herbal medication

Habitats of Chinese herbal medication are based on:

①. Soil
②. Water
③. Climate
④. Sunshine
⑤. Rainfall

Best quality herbs that come from a specific area are called "Dao Di Yao Cai" (道地药材). e.g.:

Best Ren Shen is from Northeast of China.
Best Fu Ling is from Yun Nan province.
Best Huang Lian is from Si Chuan province.
Best Di Huang is from He Nan province.
Best Er Jiao is from Shan Dong province.

2.2 Collection of Chinese medication

A. Plant origin herbs collection

Entire grass collected when their flower is in full bloom
Leaves are collected when their flowers are blooming
Flowers are collected when they are blooming
Fruits are collected when they are ripe (but some not)
roots are collected in late autumn or spring
Barks are collected in spring or early summer

B. Animal origin herbs are collected at different times.

C. Mineral origin medication herbs are collected at any time.

2.3 Storage of Chinese medication:

Preparation work for storage: to clean, dry, seal, absorb Dampness, chemical substance, reduce oxygen, increase carbon dioxide.

For extremely toxic medication, they are secured and only accessible by certain people.

3. Nomenclature of Chinese Herbal Medicine

1) **Cao** 草 means entire grass with or without root
2) **Gen** 根 means root
3) **Hua** 花 means flower
4) **Pi** 皮 means bark, peel
5) **Ren** 仁 means seed
6) **Zi** 子 means seed
7) **Shi** 石 means stone
8) **Ye** 叶 means leaf
9) **Zhi** 枝 means twig
10) **Jiao** 角 means horn
11) **Teng** 藤 means vine
12) **Tan** 碳 means charred herbs
13) **She** 蛇 means snake
14) **Zhi** 炙 means processed (As an adj.)

4. Processing of Chinese Herbal Medicine

4.1 Purpose of processing

①. Purify herbs
②. Make active components easier to dissolve
③. Increase effect
④. Remove side effects or toxicity
⑤. Change property or action
⑥. Remove unpleasant taste

4.2 Processing Method

1). Mechanical method

①. Cleaning
②. Pulverizing
③. Slicing

2). Process with Water

①. Bleaching
②. Soaking
③. Trituration with water (Shui Fei 水飞)

3). Process with Heat

①. Frying with liquid (Zhi 炙)
②. Stir-frying (Chao 炒)
   1) Stir-frying to yellow (炒黄)
   2) Stir-frying to brown(炒焦)
   3) Carbonizing（炒碳）
③. Roasting in ashes (Wei 煨)
④. Baking (Hong or Bei 烘焙)
⑤. Quick-frying (Pao 炮)
⑥. Calcining (Duan 煅)

4). Process with both Heat and water

①. Steaming (Zheng 蒸)
   a) Pure steaming
   b) Steaming with other material
②. Simmering (Ao 熬)
③. Boiling (Zhu 煮)
④. Quenching (Cui 淬)
⑤. Scalding in hot water (Tang 烫)

5). Other methods

①. Germination
②. Fermentation

5. Actions and indications of Chinese Herbal Medicine

5.1 Mechanism of the Actions of TCM medication

①. Expel pathogen and treat causes
②. Tonify Deficiency
③. Readjust function of Zhang Fu organs and meridians

5.2 Actions of TCM medication

①. To address the cause of the disease

②. To address the symptoms of the disease

6. The Properties of Chinese Herbal Medicine

6.1The Four Properties 四气

They are cool and Cold, warm and hot.

Cool or Cold, and warm or hot are only the different degrees. Cool is weaker than Cold, and warm is weaker than hot.

Herbs which are **cool or Cold** usually can **clear Heat and resolve toxicity, cool Blood, Nourish Yin and purge Fire.**

Herbs which are **warm or hot** properties can **warm the interior, dispel Cold, and tonify Yang and Qi**.

6.2 The Five Tastes 五味

A. Pungent/Acrid: expel, move Qi and Blood.

B. Sweet: tonify, harmonize, relieve spasm and pain.

C. Sour: keep, hold something to stop sweating, spontaneous emission or leukorrhagia, astringe Qi, stop bleeding and diarrhea.

D. Bitter: clear, drain to clear Heat toxicity, purge, and clear Dampness.

E. Salty: purge, soften hard masses.

F. Astringent: similar action to sour.

G. Tasteless: remove Dampness and promote urination.

6.3 Ascending and Descending, Floating and Sinking 升降浮沉

Ascending and floating: going upward or outward.

Descending and sinking: going downward and inward.

6.4 Channel Entering (Gui Jing 归经)

Each herb has a selective action on one or several channels.

6.5 Toxicity 毒性

Chinese herbal medicine can be classified into **non-toxic**（无毒）and **toxic**（有毒）according to level of toxicity. Among toxic herbs, some are slightly toxic, some are moderately toxic and others are extremely toxic.

①. Non toxic herbs 无毒 LD_{50} > 50g/kg

②. Slightly toxic herbs 小毒 LD_{50} > 50g/kg

③. Moderately toxic herbs 有毒 $LD_{50} = 6\text{-}15g/kg$

④. Extremely toxic herbs 大毒 $LD_{50} < 5g/kg$

LD50 means **M**edian **L**ethal **D**ose.

7. Herbal Combinations and Interactions

(1) Mutual accentuation (Xiang Xu 相须): herbs with similar actions reinforce each other to increase their therapeutic actions.

(2) Mutual enhancement (Xiang Shi 相使): herbs with similar actions reinforce each other, acting as principal herb and an assistant herb.

(3) Mutual conteraction (Xiang Wei 相畏): the toxicities or side effects of one herb can be reduced or eliminated by another herb.

(4) Mutual suppression (Xiang Sha 相杀): one herb reduces the side effects of another herb.

(5) Mutual antagonism (Xiang Wu 相恶): one herb reduces the therapeutic action of another herb.

(6) Mutual incompatibility (Xiang Fan 相反): two herbs used together can increase or give rise to side effect or toxicity.

(7) Single effect (Dan Xing 单行): Use the herb alone.

8. Nineteen Antagonisms and Eighteen Incompatibilities

8.1 Nineteen Antagonisms (Shi Jiu Wei)

①. Sulphur (**Liu Huang**) --- Sal Glauberis (**Mang Xiao**)

②. Hydrargyrum (**Shui Yin**) --- Arsennicum (**Pi Shuang**)

③. Radix euphorbiae (**Lang Du**) --- Lithargyrum (**Mi Tuo Seng**)

④. Crotonis Fructus (**Ba Dou**) --- Pharbitidis Semen (**Qian Niu Zi**)

⑤. Caryophylli Flos (**Ding Xiang**) --- Curcumae Radix (**Yu Jin**)

⑥. Niyrum (**Ya Xiao**) --- Rhizona Sparganii (**San Leng**)

⑦. Aconiti Radix preparata (**Wu Tou** including **Chuan Wu** and **Cao Wu**) --- Rhinocerotis Cornu (**Xi Jiao**)

⑧. Radix ginseng (**Ren Shen**) --- Trogopterori Faeces (**Wu Ling Zhi**)

⑨. Cinnamomi Cortex (**Rou Gui**) --- Halloysitum rubrum (**Chi Shi Zi**)

Translation of original Chinese saying:

1. **Liu Huang** fights **Mang Xiao**
2. **Shui Yin** should not meet **Pi Shuang**
3. **Lang Du** fears **Mi Tuo Seng**
4. **Ba Dou** does not like **Qian Niu Zi**
5. **Ding Xiang** can not meet **Yu Jin**
6. **Ya Xiao** does not cooperate with **San Leng**
7. **Chuan Wu and Cao Wu** do not work with **Xi Jiao**
8. **Ren Shen** fears **Wu Ling Zhi**
9. **Rou Gui** bullys **Chi Shi Zi**

Original saying in Chinese:

硫磺原是火中精，朴硝一见便相争，水银莫与砒霜见，狼毒最怕密陀僧，巴豆性烈最为上，偏与牵牛不顺情，丁香莫与郁金见，牙硝难合京三棱，川乌草乌不顺犀，人参最怕五灵脂，官桂善能调冷气，若逢石脂便相欺，大凡修合看顺逆，炮槛炙膊/浸莫相依。---《珍珠囊补遗药性赋》

8. 2 Eighteen Incompatibilities (Shi Ba Fan)

1). **Wu Tou** (The various forms of Radix Aconiti) is incompatible with:
  Ban Xia (Rhizoma Pinelliae Ternatae)
  Gua Lou (Fractus Trichosanthis)
  Bei Mu (Bulbus Fritillariae)
  Bai Lian (Radix Ampelopsis)
  Bai Ji (Rhizoma Bletillae Striatae)

2). **Gan Cao** (Radix Glycyrrhizae Uralensis) is incompatible with:
  Hai Zao (Herba Sargassi)
  Da Ji (Radix Euphorbiae seu Knoxiae)
  Gan Sui (Radix Euphorbiae Kansui)
  Yuan Hua (Flos Daphnes Genkwa)

3). **Li Lu (Rhizoma et Radix Veratri) is** incompatible with:
  Ren Shen (Radix Ginseng)
  Xi Yang Shen (Radix panacis Quinquefolii)
  Tai Zi Shen (Radix Pseudo-stellariae)
  Dang Shen (Radix Codonopsis Pilosulae)
  Sha Shen (Radix Adenophorae seu Glehniae)
  Dan Shen (Radix Salviae Miltiorrhiae)
  Ku Shen (Radix Sophorae Flavescentis)

Xuan Shen (Radix Scrophulariae)
Xi Xin (Herba cum Radice Asari)
Bai/Chi Shao (Yao) (Radix Paeoniae Lactiflorae)

Original saying in Chinese:
本草明言十八反，半蒌贝蔹芨攻乌，藻戟遂芫俱战草，诸参辛芍叛藜芦。--- 《珍珠囊补遗药性赋》

Pronunciation of original Chinese saying:
Ban (Xia), (Gua) **Lou**, **Bei** (Mu), (Bai) **Lian**, (Bai) **Ji** ***gong*** **Wu** (Tou);
Gong is a verb, means fight

(Hai) **Zao,** (Da) **Ji,** (Gan) **Sui**, **Yuan** (Hua), ***ju zhan*** (Gan) **Cao;**
Ju means completely. **Zhan** means fight.

Zhu Shen, (Xi) **Xin,** (Bai/Chi) **Shao** (Yao) ***pan*** **Li Lu.**
Zhu means all. **Pan** means rebel, fight.

9. Dosage of Chinese Herbal Medicine

9.1. Ancient Unit vs Modern Unit

Ancient unit: 1 Jin = 16 Liang = 160 Qian = 1600 Li
Ancient 1 Liang = modern 30g
Ancient 1 Qian = modern 3g
Ancient 1 Li = modern 0.3 g

With the exception of herbs that are toxic, strong, light or heavy, the typical dosage for most dry herbs is 3-10g a day, orally administered for adult.

9.2. Factors that Determine Dosage of Herbs

①. Property of herbs
②. Quality of herbs
③. Role of herbs in formula
④. Forms of formula
⑤. Condition of the disease
⑥. Condition of patients
⑦. Geographic and season factors
⑧. Purpose of using a certain herb

10. Administration of Chinese Herbal Medicine

10.1. Forms of Herbal Medicine

1) Decoctions (Tang 汤)
2) Pills (Wan 丸)
3) Powders (San 散)
4) Plasters (Gao 膏)
   ①. Plaster medicine (Gao Yao 膏药)
   ②. Herbal patch (Tie Gao 贴膏)
5) Ointment (Ran Gao 软膏)
6) Vermilion pills (Dan 丹)
7) Herbal wines (Yao Jiu 药酒)

10.2. Decocting Method

1) Utensils for decocting
2) Water
3) Type of Heat and decocting time
   Military Fire (wu huo 武火)
   Civilian Fire (wen huo 文火).
4) Most formulas need to be decocted for 20-30 minutes.
5) Special methods for decocting
   ①. Decocted early (Xian Jian 先煎)
   ②. Added later (Hou Xia 后下)
   ③. Wrapped in gauze (Bao Jian 包煎)
   ④. Separately decocted (Ling Jian 另煎 or Ling Dun 另炖
   ⑤. Dissolved in hot decoction (Yang Hua 烊化)
   ⑥. Taken with the hot decoction (Chong Fu 冲服)
   ⑦. Use decoction as water
   ⑧. Boiled powders (Zhu San 煮散)

10.3 Times of Decocting

Most formulas are decocted two to three times.

10.4. Administration Method

A. Time of administration
   ①. Taken on an empty Stomach: to kill parasites, relieve food stagnation or drain downward

②. Taken before meals: for treating Stomach or intestinal diseases is beneficial for the maximum absorption.
③. Taken after a meal: with herbs that irritate the Stomach.
④. Taken before bedtime: to calm the spirit.
⑤. Taken at a certain time: for malaria.
⑥. Taken immediately: in emergency situation.

B. Frequency of taking

A daily dosage can be divided into two or three portions to be taken throughout the day. For serious or acute conditions, herbs can be taken every four hours until the patient's condition improves.

11.Special consideration of Herbal Treatment

①. Herbal treatment during pregnancy.
②. Herbal treatment during breast feeding.
③. Herbal treatment for neonatal and pediatric patients.
④. Herbal treament for geriatric patients.
⑤. Herbal taboo with food (dietetic restraint)

Practice 1

1. The Cold nature herbs have the functions of
A. Dispersing Cold, clearing Heat, purging Fire
B. Tonifying Yang, dispersing Cold, restoring the collapse of Yang
C. Clearing Heat, removing toxins, nourishing Yin
D. Restoring the collapse of Yang, warming up the interior, removing toxin

2. Four properties (Si Qi, 四气) refer to:
A. Cold, Cool; Hot, Warm;
B. Sour, Sweet, Bitter, Salty;
C. Spring, Summer, Autumn, Winter;
D. Rising, falling, floating, sinking;

3. Five flavors (tastes) refer to:
A. Sour (suan); Sweet (gan); Bitter (ku); Salty (xian) and Pungent acrid (xin);
B. Sour (suan); tasteless (dan); Bitter (ku); Pungent (xin) and astringent (se)
C. Sour (suan); Sweet (gan); Bitter (ku); Salty (xian) and Tastless (dan);
D. Sour (suan); astringent (se); Bitter (ku); Salty (xian) and Pungent acrid (xin);

4. The herbs of same taste generally have similar effects; different taste, different effects.
A. Yes
B. No

5. The purpose of processing herbs is:
A. To eliminate or minimize toxicity and side effects; increase potency.
B. To alter the properties and functions of herbs in order to meet therapeutic needs.
C. To facilitate decoction, preparation and storage;
D. To clean and to remove odor.
E. All of the above.

6. If a patient complains of coughing due to rebellious Lung Qi, no Cold, no Heat, which of the following herbs is the best to use?
A. The herb which has a bitter taste, neutral in the properties anddirecting downward in action
B. The herb which has a pungent taste, hot properties and floating in action

C. The herb which has a sweet taste, Cold properties and floating in action
D. The herb which has a bitter taste, hot properties and rising in action

7. If a patient has an Exterior syndrome (or external pathogens in the surface of the body), which of the following herbs will you use?
A. The herb which is rising
B. The herb which is lowering
C. The herb which is floating
D. The herb which is sinking

8. Warm nature herbs have the function of
A. Dispersing Cold, clearing Heat, purging Fire
B. Warming the interior, dispeling Cold, and tonifying Yang and Qi
C. Clearing Heat, removing toxin, nourishing yin
D. Restoring the collapse of Yang, clearing Heat, removing Fire-toxin

9. "Two herbs are used in combination, toxicity or side effects may result" refers to
A. Mutual assistance
B. Mutual restraint
C. Mutual detoxification
D. Incompatibility

10. If Sheng Jiang (fresh ginger) can reduce or remove the toxic property of Sheng Ban Xia (pinellia), the relationship is called
A. Mutual assistance
B. Incompatibility
C. Mutual detoxication
D. Mutual Inhibition

11. All of the following compatibility can be used in clinic EXCEPT
A. Mutual assistance
B. Mutual restraint
C. Mutual detoxication
D. Incompatibility

12. Ding Xiang (Clove flower bud) is antagonistic with
A. San Leng (Scirpus)

B. Ren Shen (Ginseng)
C. Yu Jin (Turmeric Tuber)
D. Chi Shi Zhi (Halloysite)

13. Ku Shen (Sophora root) is incompatible with
A. Ren Shen (Ginseng root)
B. Gan Cao (Licorice root)
C. Wu Tou (Aconite)
D. Li Lu (Veratrum root)

14. What kind of herb is contraindicated for pregnant women?
A. Tonifying herb
B. Relieving Exterior herb
C. Toxic herb
D. Warm herb

15. Ban Xia (pinellia rhizome) is incompatible with
A. Bei Mu (Fritillaria Bulb.)
B. Bai Ji (Bletilla Rhizome)
C. Wu Tou (Aconite)
D. Gan Cao(Licorice root)

16. Xi Xin (Asarum) is incompatible with
A. Ren Shen (Ginseng root)
B. Gan Cao (Licorice root)
C. Wu Tou (Aconite)
D. Li Lu (Veratrum root)

17. Ren Shen (Ginseng) is antagonistic with
A. Wu Ling Zhi (flying squirrel feces)
B. Gan Cao (Licorice root)
C. Rou Gui (Cinnamon bark)
D. Chi Shi Zhi (Halloysite or Kaolin)

18. "Herbs of similar characteristics and functions are used in coordination to strengthen their effects" is called
A. Mutual detoxication
B. Mutual reinforcement

C. Mutual restraint
D. Mutual incompatible

19. Using Huang Qi (radix astragali membranacei) as a chief herb and Fu Ling (Sclerotium Poriae Cocos) as a deputy herb to tonify qi and promote urination is an example of?
A. Mutual antagonism
B. Mutual counteraction
C. Mutual enhancement
D. Mutual incompatibility

20. 1 Qian equals
A. 30 grams
B. 10 Liang
C. 3 grams
D. 0.3 grams

Answer Key: 1C. 2A. 3A. 4A. 5E. 6A. 7C. 8B. 9D. 10C. 11D. 12C. 13D. 14C. 15C. 16D. 17A. 18B. 19C. 20C

Chapter 1 Herbs that Release the Exterior

1. Common characteristics:

①. All of them are acrid/pungent.

②. Most of them go to LU or BL channel.

③. Most of them have diaphoretic, antipyretic, analgesic, antibiotic, and antivirus actions

④. Some of them have additional functions: stops cough and wheezing, controls pain or spasms, and vents rashes such as measles.

2. Symptom Exterior Syndrome:

Chill, fever, headache, stiff neck, general muscle ache and/or sweat, runny nose.

3. Causes of Exterior Syndrome:

Wind-Heat;
Wind-Cold;
Wind-Dampness;
Summer-Heat;

4. Common Contraindications:

①. Yin Deficiency

②. Spontaneous sweating

③. Night sweating

④. Chronic boils and carbuncles

⑤. Lin syndrome

⑥. Blood loss

5. Cautions:

①. Stop taking when desired effect is obtained.

②. Should not be decocted longer.

Section 1 Warm, Pungent Herbs that Release the Exterior

1. Ma Huang　Herba Ephedrae　（麻黄）
2. Gui Zhi　Ramulus Cinnamomi　（桂枝）
3. Zi Su　Folium et Caulis Perillae　（紫苏）
4. Sheng Jiang　Rhizoma Zingiberis Recens　（生姜）
5. Jing Jie　Herba Schizonepetae　（荆芥）
6. Fang Feng　Radix Ledebouriellae　（防风）
7. Bai Zhi　Radix Angelicae Dahuricae　（白芷）
8. Xi Xin　Radix et Rhizoma Asari　（细辛）
9. Qiang Huo　Rhizoma et Radix Notopterygii　（羌活）
10. Gao Ben　Rhizoma et Radix Ligustici　（藁本）
11. Xiang Ru　Herba Moslae　（香薷）
12. Cang Er Zi　Xanthii Fructus　（苍耳子）
13. Xin Yi Hua　Flos Magnoliae　（辛夷花）
14. Cong Bai　Bulbus Allii Fistulosi　（葱白）

Name	Property	CN	Actions & Indications	Remarks
Ma Huang (Herba Ephedrae) 麻黄 Ephedra stem, Ma-huang	Pungent slightly bitter warm	LU BL	1. **Induce sweating and release the Exterior:** for Exterior Wind-Cold syndrome *without sweating* (Wind-Cold Excess syndrome); usually used with Gui Zhi as in Ma Huang Tang. 2. **Disseminate Lung Qi, calm wheezing:** for cough and wheezing due to Lung Qi being obstructed; usually used with Xin Ren as in San Ao Tang. 3. **Promotes urination and reduces edema:** for edema with Exterior condition. A) General edema with Exterior Wind syndrome; used with Shi Gao, Gan Can,	3-10g Contraindicated with hyper-thyroidism, hypertension，angina pectoris and insomnia. **Sheng Ma Huang**:(not processed by honey) is good for inducing sweating. **Zhi Ma Huang**: (honey processed) is good for calming

			Sheng Jiang (such as Yue Pi Tang). B) Edema with deep pulse and Cold condition; used with Fu Zi, Gan Cao. (such as Ma Huang Fu Zi Gan Cao Tang)	wheezing.
Gui Zhi (Cinnamomi Ramulus) 桂枝 Cinnamon twig, Cassia twig	Pungent sweet warm	LU BL HT	1. **Induces sweating and releases the Exterior:** mainly for Exterior Wind-Cold *with sweating* (Wind-Cold Deficiency syndrome) as in Gui Zhi Tang. 2. **Unblocks and warms channels:** for abdominal Cold pain, dysmenorrhea, amenorrhea due to Cold that cause Blood stasis. for Bi syndrome due to Wind-Cold-Damp. A) With Yang Deficiency; used with Fu Zi (such as Gui Zhi Fu Zi Tang) B) With Blood Deficiency; used with Bai Shao, Huang Qi (such as Huang Qi Gui Zhi Wu Wu Tang). C) For Blood stasis, amenorrhea, abdominal pain and abdominal mass; used with Fu Ling (Gui Zhi Fu Ling Wan). D) For abdominal pain due to Cold syndrome of Deficiency type in the middle-Jiao; used with Huang Qi (Huang Qi Jian Zhong Tang). 3. **Warms Yang Qi:** for (1) edema due to Kidney Yang	3-10g

			Deficiency, (2) chest pain due to chest Yang Deficiency leading to Blood stasis, (3) Heart and Spleen Yang Deficiency leading to water retention, and (4) palpitation, arhythmia due to Heart Yang Deficiency. A) For deficient Yang of Heart and Spleen; used with Fu Ling, Bai Zhu (Ling Gui Zhu Gan Tang) B) For dysfunction of Qi activities of bladder; used with Fu Ling, Ze Xie (Wu Ling San). C) For chest pain; used with Xie Bai, Zhi Shi. D) For palpitation, slow pulse with irregular intervals; used with Zhi Gan Can, Ren Shen. (such as Zhi Gan Can Tang).	
Zi Su (Folium et Caulis Perillae) 紫苏 Perilla leaf	Pungent aromatic warm	LU SP	1. **Induces sweating and release the Exterior:** for Exterior Wind-Cold syndrome; used with Xing Ren, Qian Hu (such as Xing Su San). 2. **Moves Qi and expands the middle:** for nausea, vomiting, poor appetite, restless fetus and morning sickness. A) For Cold; used with Hou Po. B) For Heat; used with Huang Lian.	3-10g The leaf of it is called **Zi Su Ye** and is good for inducing sweating. The slender stalk of it is called **Zi Su Geng** or **Su Geng** and is good for calming fetus.

			C) For Phlegm; used with Ban Xia, Hou Po. 3. **Releases seafood poisoning:** for abdominal pain, vomiting due to seafood poisoning. Singlely used 30-60g or used with Sheng Jiang.	
Sheng Jiang (Zingiberis Rhizoma Recens) 生姜 Fresh giner rhizome	Pungent warm	LU SP ST	1. **Dispels Cold and releases the Exterior:** for Exterior Wind Cold syndrome; used with red sugar or Gui Zhi, Bai Shao, Gan Cao (such as Gui Zhi Tang). 2. **Warms Middle Jiao and stops vomiting:** for vomiting due to any cause, best for vomiting due to Stomach Cold. It is one of the best herbal medicines for vomiting. Also for Stomachache due to Middle Jiao Coldness. 3. **Warms up Lung and stops cough:** for cough due to Wind-Cold or Phlegm. 4. **Resolves toxicity:** for toxicity due to food poisoning or overdose of other herbs such as Ban Xia (Pinelliae Rhizoma) and Tian Nan Xing. For fish and crab poisoning; used with Zi Su Ye.	3-10g
Jing Jie (Schizonepetae) 荆芥 Schizonepeta stem or bud	Pungent Aromatic **slightly warm**	LU LR	1. **Releases the Exterior and expels Wind:** for either Wind-Cold or Wind-Heat syndromes. A) Wind-Cold syndrome;	3-10g

			used with Fang Feng, Qiang Huo (such as Jing Fang Bai Du San). B) Wind-Heat syndrome-with Yin Hua, Lian Qiao, Bo He. (such as Yin Qiao San). 2. **Vents rashes and stops itching:** for the early stage of measles and pruritic skin eruptions; used with Bo He. 3. **Stops bleeding:** as an auxiliary herb for hemorrhage by having the herb charred. Used with Ce Bai Ye, Zong Lu Tan. 4. Also for early stage boils and carbuncles with Exterior syndrome.	
Fang Feng (Saposhnikoviae Radix) 防风 Ledebouriella root, Siler	Pungent sweet warm	BL LR SP	1. **Expels Wind and releases the Exterior:** for all kind of Wind-Cold syndromes. A) Wind-Cold syndrome ; used with Jing Jie. B) Wind-Heat syndrome ; used with Bo He, Lian Qiao. 2. **Expels Wind-Dampness and alleviates pain:** for Bi syndrome especially when Wind predominates; used with Qiang Huo, Du Huo (such as Juan Pi Tang). 3. **Expels inner Wind and relieves spasm:** for trembling and tetany due to Wind toxicity invasion; used with Bai Fu Zi, Tian Ma (such as Yu Zhen San).	3-10g It is for all Wind syndromes, hot or Cold, upper or lower, Exterior or interior.

			4. It also goes to Liver and Spleen channels for Liver Qi stagnation overacting Spleen manifested as abdominal pain following diarrhea, after diarrhea pain reduced.	
Bai Zhi (Angelicae Dahuricae Radix) 白芷 Angelica root, Chinese Angelica root	Pungent warm	LU ST	**1. Releases the Exterior, expels Wind-Cold,:** for Wind-Cold syndrome. Good at stopping pain and opening nasal orifice due to Wind-Cold. A) Wind-Cold; used with Fang Feng, Qiang Huo (such as Jiu Wei Qiang Huo Tang). B) Wind-Heat; used with Lian Qiao, Bo He. **2. Expels Wind and stops pain:** for headache, toothache, Bi syndrome. Good at Yangming /frontal headache with supraorbital bone pain. A) Headache especially in the forehead; used with Ju Hua, Chuan Xiong (such as Chuan Xiong Cha Tiao San). B) Headache due to stuffy nose ; used with Cang Er Zi, Xin Yi Hua (such as Cang Er Zi San). **3. Opens nasal orifice**: for Bi Yuan (Nasal disorder) manifested as running nose, nasal congestion with headache; used with Cang Er Zi, Xin Yi Hua (such as Cang Er Zi San). **4. Expels Dampness:** for excessive vaginal discharge	3-10g **Side effect:** BP increase, drooling, convulsion.

			due to Cold Dampness; used with Bai Zhu, Fu Ling, Che Qian Zi. 5. **Reduces swelling and expels pus:** for early stages superficial sores and carbuncle. A) Mastitis; used with Bei Mu, Pu Gong Ying. B) Sores and swellings; used with Yin Hua.	
Xi Xin (Asari Herba) 细辛 Chinese wild ginger, Asarum	Pungent Warm **Toxic**	LU KI	1. **Disperses Cold and releases the Exterior:** for Exterior Wind Cold syndrome with body ache, especially with Dampness or underlying Yang Deficiency; used with Ma Huang, Fu Zi (such as Ma Huang Fu Zi Xi Xin). 2. **Dispels Wind and relieves pain:** for headache, toothache and Bi syndrome due to Wind Cold; used with Qiang Huo, Fang Feng, Bai Zhi. 3. **Opens orifice:** for Bi Yuan (Nasal disorder) manifested as running nose, nasal congestion with headache, and loss of consciousness. 4. **Warms up Lung and transforms thin mucus:** for cough and wheezing due to Exterior Wind-Cold and interior Cold Phlegm; used with Gan Jiang, Ban Xia, Wu Wei Zi (such as Xiao Qing Long Tang).	**1-3g in decoction and 0.5-1g as powder. Incompatible with Li Lu** Over dosage can be poisonous manifested as headache, vomiting, irritability, sweating, rigidity of neck, thirst, body temperature and BP increasing, dilated puples, hot flush in early stage, then convulsion, loss of consciousness, finally death due to respiratory failure.
Qiang Huo	Pungent	BL	1. **Expels Wind-Cold to release**	3-10g

(Notopterygii Rhizoma seu Radix) 羌活 Notopterygium root, Chiang-huo	bitter aromatic warm	KI	**the Exterior:** for Wind-Cold syndrome, especially headache and bodyache due to Wind Cold with Dampness; used with Fang Feng, Bai Zhi, Xi Xin (such as Jiu Wei Qiang Huo Tang). 2. **Expels Wind-Dampness and stops pain:** for Bi syndrome, especially in the upper part of the body; used with Du Huo, Fang Feng, Wei Ling Xian (such as Qiang Huo Shen Shi Tang).	It can guide Qi to the TaiYang and Du channel. Overdosage can cause vomiting.
Gao Ben (Ligustici Rhizoma) 藁本 Chinese lovage root, ligusticum root, kao-pen	Pungent warm	BL	1. **Expels Wind-Cold:** for Wind-Cold syndrome, especially with headache and nasal congestion (TaiYang Wind-Cold). 2. **Expels Wind-Dampness and stops pain:** for Bi syndrome due to Wind-Cold-Dampness; used with Chuan Xiong, Qiang Huo (such as Qiang Huo Sheng Shi Tang).	3-10g
Xiang Ru (Moslae Herba) 香薷 Aromatic Madder, Elsholtzia	Pungent Aromatic slightly warm	LU ST	1. **Induces sweating and releases the Exterior:** for Wind-Cold *during the summer*, especially when accompanied by Dampness; used with Bian Dou, Hou Po (such as Xiang Ru San). 2. **Promotes urination and reduces swelling:** for edema and urinary difficulty, especially associated with an Exterior syndrome; used alone or with Bai Zhu.	3-10g It is called "the summer Ma Huang (ephedra)".

Cang Er Zi (Xanthii Fructus) 苍耳子 Cocklebur fruit, Xanthium	Pungent bitter warm **Toxic**	LU	1. **Expels Wind and releases the Exterior:** for Exterior disorders with a splitting headache that radiates to the back of the neck, as an auxiliary herb. 2. **Opens nasal passages:** for any nasal or sinus problem with a thick, viscous discharge and related headache; used with Xin Yi Hua, Bai Zhi (such as Cang Er Zi San). 3. **Dispels Wind-Dampness:** for Bi syndrome; used alone or with Wei Ling Xian, Rou Gui. 4. **Kills parasites:** for skin disorders with itching.	3-10g
Xin Yi (Hua) (Magnoliae Flos) 辛夷(花) Magnolia flower	Pungent warm	LU ST	1. **Dispels Wind and releases the Exterior:** for Exterior Wind Cold syndrome. 2. **Unblocks nasal passages:** for running nose, nasal obstruction or congestion, loss of smell, sinusitis, or nasal related headache. A) Cold syndrome, with Fang Feng, Xi Xin, Bai Zhi. B) Heat syndrome, with Bo He, Huang Qin.	3-10g **wrapped** It is good at unblocking nasal orifice.
Cong Bai (Allii Fistulosi) Bulbus 葱白 Scallion or spring onion	Pungent warm	LU ST	1. **Induces sweating and releases the Exterior:** for early stage external Wind-Cold syndrome; used with Dou Chi (such as Cong Chi Tang) 2. **Disperses Cold and unblocks Yang Qi:** for abdominal pain	3-10g

			and distention, or nasal congestion due to blockage of Yang Qi caused by Cold; used with Fu Zi, Gan Jiang (such as Bai Tong Tang). 3. **Resolves toxicity and disperses clumps**: for sores and abscesses.	

Practice 2

1. Ma Huang (Ephedra stem)'s flavor and nature (i.e., temperature) are:
A. Acrid, slightly bitter and warm
B. Acrid, slightly bitter and neutral
C. Acrid, slightly sweet and warm
D. Acrid, sweet and cool

2. Ma Huang (Ephedra stem) mainly treats:
A. Wind Cold Exterior Excess syndrome
B. Wind Heat Exterior Excess syndrome
C. Exterior deficient Wind Cold syndrome
D. Exterior deficient Wind Heat syndrome

3. Besides resolving the Exterior, Gui Zhi (Cinnamon Twig) also:
A. Harmonizes the constructive and defensive
B. Warms the channels and scatters Cold
C. Frees the flow of Yang and transforms the Qi
D. All of the above.

4. Which of the following herb should be used to treat Wind-Cold Deficiency with sweating, aversion to Wind, and emission of the Heat?
A. Ma Huang (Ephedra stem)
B. Gui Zhi (Cinnamon twig)
C. Fang Feng(Radix Ledebouriellae Divaricatae)
D. Su Ye (Perilla leaf)

5. Which Exterior-resolver expels Wind, out-thrusts rashes, and stops bleeding?
A. Zi Su Ye (Perilla leaf)
B. Jing Jie (Schizonepeta stem or bud)
C. Sheng Jiang (Rhizoma Zingiberis)
D. Ma Huang (Ephedra stem)

6. Which herbs can expel Wind, remove Dampness to relieve pain, extinguish internal Wind to relieve spasm?
A. Jing Jie (Schizonepeta stem or bud)

B. Fang Feng (Ledebouriella root or Siler)
C. Bai Zhi (Angelica root)
D. Xi Xin (Chinese Wild Ginger)

7. Which of the following are actions of Qiang Huo (Rhizoma et notopterygii)?
A. Releases Exterior and expels Wind, Expel Wind Damp and relieves pain, Stops internal Wind
B. Releases Exterior and expels Wind Cold, Relieves back pain from Wind Cold invasion
C. Releases Exterior and expels Cold, Unblocks obstructions and relieves pain, Guides Qi to Tai Yang and Du channels
D. Releases Exterior and expels Cold, Warms the middle and stops vomiting, Expels Cold and stops cough, Regulates Ying and Wei

8. What is the regular dosage for Xi Xin (Asari Herba)?
A. No more than 1 Qian
B. No more than 2 Qian
C. No more than 3 Qian
D. No more than 4 Qian

9. Which herb is also known as "Summer Ma Huang"?
A. Sheng Jiang (Fresh Ginger Rhizome)
B. Chai Hu (Radix Bupleuri)
C. Xiang Ru (Moslae Herba)
D. Zi Su Ye (Perilla Leaf)

10. Jing Jie and Fang Feng both
A. Disperse Wind and relieve the Exterior
B. Disperse Wind and eliminate Dampness
C. Disperse Wind and brighten the eyes
D. Disperse Wind and transforms Phlegm

11. Sheng Jiang (Fresh Ginger Rhizome) is best for stopping which pattern of vomiting:
A. Stomach Deficiency
B. Stomach Heat
C. Qi stagnation
D. Stomach Cold

12. Which herb dispels Wind, scatters Cold, and opens the orifice of the nose?
A. Zi Su Ye (Perilla Leaf)
B. Sheng Jiang (Fresh Ginger Rhizome)
C. Xin Yi Hua (Flos Manoliae Liliflorae)
D. Fang Feng (Ledebouriella root)

13. Which of the following statement is correct?
A. Sheng Ma Huang (unprepared, without honey processed) is good at inducing sweating, while Zhi Ma Huang (prepared, Honey processed) is good at cough and calming wheezing.
B. Gui Zhi (Cinnamon Twig) is contraindicated in deficient Yin with Heat signs.
C. Ma Huang (Ephedra Stem) is contraindicated for hyperthyroidism, hypertension, angina pectoris and insomnia.
D. All of above

14. Which of the following statement is correct?
A. Zi Su Ye (Perilla Leaf) can used for abdominal pain, vomiting due to seafood poisoning. It can be used singly up to 30-60g for resolving poisoning.
B. Fang Feng (Radix Ledebouriellae Divaricatae) goes to Liver and Spleen channels, can be used for Liver Qi stagnation overacting Spleen manifested as abdominal pain following diarrhea, after diarrhea pain reduced.
C. Qiang Huo (notopterygium root) with overdosage can cause vomiting.
D. All of above

15. Which of the following statement is correct?
A. Qiang Huo (notopterygium root) is good for Yang Ming Headache.
B. Gao Ben (Chinese lovage root, ligusticum root, kao-pen) is good for Shao Yang Headache.
C. Bai Zhi (Angelica root) is good for Yang Ming Headache.
D. Xi Xin (Chinese wild ginger) is good for Tai Yang Headache.

16. Which of the following herbs is toxic?
A. Xi Xin (Chinese Wild Ginger)
B. Cang Er Zi (Cocklebur Fruit, Xanthium)
C. Neither of them
D. Both of them

17. Which of the following statement is NOT correct?
A. Sheng Jiang (Fresh ginger Rhizome) can resolve toxicity due to food poisoning or treating the effects of overdose of other herbs such as Ban Xia (Pineliae Rhizoma) and Tian Nan Xing.
B. Sheng Jiang (Fresh ginger Rhizome) is one of the best herbal medicines for vomiting.
C. Cong Bai (scallion or spring onion) can be used for either abdominal pain and distention or nasal congestion due to blockage of Yang Qi by Cold.
D. Cang Er Zi (Cocklebur fruit, Xanthium) with overdosage can lead to vomiting, abdominal pain, diarrhea.
E. None of them

Answers Keys: 1A. 2A. 3D. 4B. 5B. 6B. 7C. 8A. 9C. 10A. 11D. 12C. 13D. 14D. 15C. 16D.17E

Section 2 Cool, Pungent Herbs that Release the Exterior

1. Bo He (Herba Menthae) 薄荷
2. Niu Bang Zi (Fructus Arctii) 牛蒡子
3. Chan Tui (Periostracum Cicadae) 蝉蜕
4. Sang Ye (Folium Mori) 桑叶
5. Ju Hua (Flos Chrysanthemi) 菊花
6. Chai Hu (Radix Bupleuri) 柴胡
7. Sheng Ma (Rhizoma Cimicifugae) 升麻
8. Ge Gen (Radix Puerariae) 葛根
9. Man Jing Zi (Fructus Viticis) 蔓荆子
10. Dan Dou Chi (Semen Sojae Praeparatum) 淡豆豉
11. Fu Ping (Herba Spirodelae) 浮萍
12. Mu Zei (Herba Equiseti Hiemalis) 木贼

Name	Property	CN	Actions & Indications	Remarks
Bo He (Menthae Haplocalycis Herba) 薄荷 Field Mint, Mentha	Pungent Aromatic Cool	LU LR	1. **Expels Wind-Heat:** for Wind-Heat syndrome with fever, cough, headache, red eyes, and sore throat due to Wind Heat; used with Jin Yin Hua, Lian Qiao (such as Yin Qiao San). 2. **Clears head, eyes and throat:** for headache, red eyes, lacrimation and sore throat; used with Ju Hua, Niu Bang Zi, Huang Qin. 3. **Soothes Liver Qi:** for hypochondriac distention, emotional instability, menstruation disorder due to Liver Qi stagnation; used with Chai Hu, Xiang Fu. 4. **Vents rashes:** for early stages measles; used with Ge Gen, Sheng Ma, Niu Bang Zi. 5. **Expels turbid filth:** for Summer	**3-6g**. Decoct it later.

			Heat gastric disturbance (Sha Zhang) with abdominal pain, vomiting, diarrhea.	
Niu Bang Zi (Arctii Fructus) 牛蒡子 Great Burdock fruit or Arctium	Pungent Bitter Cold	LU ST	1. **Expels Wind-Heat:** for fever, sore throat, cough due to Wind-Heat; used with Bo He, Jin Yin Hua, Lian Qiao (such as Yin Qiao San) 2. **Benefits throat:** for sore, red, swollen throat due to Wind-Heat. 3. **Resolves toxicity:** for carbuncles, erythemas, and mumps due to Heat toxicity. 4. **Moistens Intestine:** for sore throat, rashes with constipation 5. **Vents rashes:** for acute febrile maculopapule, rashes, mumps due to Heat toxicity.	6-12g
Chan Tui (Cicadae Periostracum) 蝉蜕 Cicada moulting	Sweet Cold	LU LR	1. **Expels Wind-Heat:** for chills and fever, loss of voice and swollen, sore throat due to Wind-Heat; used with Bo He, Lian Qiao. 2. **Clears eyes:** red, painful, and swollen eyes due to Wind-Heat, or blurry vision, superficial visual obstruction; used with Ju Hua. 3. **Stops spasm and extinguishes Wind:** for childhood febrile diseases with convulsions, spasms, delirium due to Wind, or night terrors; used with Bai Ji Li, Jing Jie, Fang Feng. 4. **Vents rashes:** for early stage of measles with an incomplete expression of the rash; used with Ge Gen, Niu Bang Zi, Lian Qiao.	3-10g Contraindicated for pregnancy because it can reduce sperm count and deform the fetus;
Sang Ye Mori Folium	Sweet Bitter	LU LR	1. **Expels Wind-Heat:** for externally contracted Wind-Heat with fever,	5-10g

桑叶 Mulberry leaf	Cold		headache, sore throat, and cough; used with Ju Hua, Bo He, Lu Gen (such as Sang Ju Yin). **2. Calms Liver and clears the eyes:** for red, sore, dry or painful eyes, or spots in front of the eyes, vertigo. A) Due to excessive Heat or Wind-Heat in the Liver channel, used with Jue Ming Zi, Ju Hua. B) Due to Liver Yin Deficiency, used with Ma Zi Ren. **3. Clears Lung and moistens Dryness:** for Lung Dryness with cough, and dry mouth or Lung Heat with thick, yellow sputum; used with Xing Ren, Bei Mu, Mai Men Dong such as Sang Xing Tang). **4. Cools Blood and stops bleeding**	
Ju Hua Chrysanthemi Flos 菊花 Chrysanthemum flower	Pungent Sweet Bitter Slightly Cold	LU LR	**1. Expels Wind-Heat:** for Wind-Heat with fever and headache, cough; used with Sang Ye, Lian Qiao, Bo He (such as Sang Ju Yin). **2. Clears the eyes:** for red, swollen, dry, and/or painful eyes, spots in front of the eyes, blurry vision. A) Due to Wind-Heat in Liver channel or flaming up of Liver Fire; used with Sang Ye. B) Due to Deficiency of Liver Yin and Kidney Yin; used with Shu Di, Shan Yao, Shan Zhu Yu (such as Qi Ju Di Huang Wan). **3. Subdues Liver Yang and extinguishes Wind:** for dizziness,	10-15g

			headache, and deafness due to Liver Yang rising; used with Bai Shao, Mu Li. 4. **Resolves toxicity:** for toxic sores and swellings.	
Chai Hu (Bupleuri Radix) 柴胡 Thorowax root, bupleurum, Chinese thorowax root	Bitter Pungent Cool	GB LR PC SJ	1. **Releases the Exterior and reduces fever:** for fever due to Wind-Heat or Wind-Cold, alternating chill and fever with bitter taste, flank pain, irritability, vomiting, and a stifling sensation in the chest related with ShaoYang disorders. Also treats malaria; used with Ban Xia, Sheng Jiang, Huang Qin (such as Xiao Chai Hu Tang). 2. **Soothes Liver Qi:** for Liver Qi stagnation with dizziness, vertigo, chest and flank pain, emotional instability, or menstrual problems; used with Shao Yao, Zhi Ke, Gan Cao (such as Si Ni San). 3. **Raises Yang Qi:** for inner organ prolapse, hemorrhoids, excessive vaginal discharge, bleeding or exhaustion; used with Huang Qi, Shen Ma (such as Bu Zhong Yi Qi Tang).	3-10g
Sheng Ma (Cimicifugae Rhizoma) 升麻 Black cohosh rhizome, Bugbane rhizome cimicifuga	Slightly Sweet Pungent Cool	LI LU SP	1. **Expels Wind-Heat and releases the muscles:** for headache due to Exterior Wind-Heat or the early stages of measles; used with Ge Gen. 2. **Clears Heat toxicity:** for mouth sore, toothache, swollen or painful gums, ulcerated lips or gums, painful and swollen throat due to Wind Heat; used with Shi Gao,	3-10g

			Huang Lian (such as Qing Wei San). **3. Raises Yang Qi and lifts sinking:** for shortness of breath, fatigue, and organ prolapse due to Middle Jiao Qi sinking. Also used for guiding the other herbs going upward; used with Huang Qi, Bai Zhu, Chen Pi (such as Bu Zhong Yi Qi Tang).	
Ge Gen (Puerariae Radix) 葛根 Kudzu root or Pueraria	Sweet Acrid Cool	SP ST	**1. Expels Wind-Heat and releases the muscles:** for Exterior disorders lodged in the muscles manifesting in fever, headache, and stiff or tight upper back and neck. A) Due to Wind-Heat with internal Heat; used with Huang Qin, Chai Hu. B) Due to Wind-Cold; used with Ma Huang, Gui Zhi, Bai Shao (Ge Gen Tang). **2. Relieves Heat and generates fluids:** for thirst due to Stomach Heat, especially suitable in cases of externally contracted Heat. **3. Vents measles:** to hasten recovery from measles with incomplete expression of the rash; used with Sheng Ma. **4. Raises Yang Qi and stops diarrhea:** for diarrhea or dysenteric disorders due to Heat. Can also be used for diarrhea due to Spleen Deficiency, when combined with appropriate herbs; used with Huang Qin, Huang	10-15g Good at upper back and neck stiffness caused by Wind

			Lian. **5. Reduces Blood pressure:** for headache, dizziness, tinnitus, or parenthesis that is related hypertension.	
Man Jing Zi (Viticis Fructus) 蔓荆子 Vitex fruit seed	Bitter Pungent Bitter Cool	BL LR ST	**1. Expels Wind-Heat:** for Exterior Wind-Heat, especially with headache or eye pain; used with Chuan Xiong, Ju Hua. **2. Clears eyes:** for Liver channel Wind-Heat manifesting as excessive tearing, red, painful, or swollen eyes, or spots in front of the eyes; used with Ju Hua, Bai Ji Li. **3. Drains Wind Dampness:** as an auxiliary herb for Wind-Dampness Bi syndrome with limbs stiffness, numbness, cramping or heaviness; used with Fang Feng, Du Huo.	5-10g Also for sciatica, constipation, cataract, insomnia, gastritis.
Dan Dou Chi (Sojae Semen preparatum) 淡豆鼓 Prepared soybean	Pungent Sweet Cool	LU ST	**1. Expels Wind:** for both Wind Heat and Wind Cold Exterior disorders. A) Wind Heat; used with Jin Yin Hua, Lian Qiao, Niu Bang Zi (such as Yin Qiao San). B) Wind Cold; used with Cong Bai (such as Cong Chi Tang). **2. Eliminates irritability:** for irritability, restlessness, stifling sensation in the chest and insomnia after febrile disorder; used with Zhi Zi (such as Zhi Zi Chi Tang).	10-15g Contraindicated for nursing mother.
Fu Ping (Spirodelae Herba) 浮萍	Pungent Cold	BL LU	**1. Induces sweating and expels Wind-Heat:** for Exterior Heat with headache and body aches without sweating. It is one of the	3-10g

Duckweed, Spirodela			few cool, acrid herbs that induce sweating; used with Bo He, Lian Qiao, Jing Jie or use alone. **2. Vents rashes and stops itching:** for hastening the full expression of measles to accelerate resolution of the disease. Also used for Wind rash; used with Niu Bang Zi, Bo He. **3. Promotes urination:** for hot superficial edema primarily affecting the upper body with urinary difficulty.	
Mu Zei (Equiseti Hiemalis Herba) 木贼 Scouring rush; shave grass	Sweet Bitter Neutral	LU LR	**1. Expels Wind-Heat, clears the eyes:** for Wind-Heat affecting the eyes and causes redness, pain, swelling, cloudiness, blurred vision, pterygium, or excessive tearing. with Ju Hua. **2. Clears Heat and stops bleeding:** as an auxiliary herb for Blood in the stool or hemorrhoids; used with Huang Qin, Di Yu.	3-10g

Practice 3

1. In addition to resolving the Exterior and clearing Heat, Bo He (Field mint):
A. Clears the head and eyes
B. Out-thrusts rashes
C. Course the Liver and resolves depression
D. All of above.

2. Which of the following herb is not acrid and warm?
A. Ma Huang (Ephedra stem)
B. Gui Zhi (Cinnamon twig)
C. Zi Su Ye (Perilla leaf)
D. Bo He (Field mint, Mentha)

3. Which of the following herbs can disperse Wind-Heat, benefit throat, resolve toxicity, vent rashes and moisten the Intestines?
A. Bo He (Herba Menthae)
B. Niu Bang Zi (Fructus Arctii)
C. Chan Tui (Periostracum Cicadae)
D. Sang Ye (Folium Mori)

4. Which of the following herbs can treat chills and fever, loss of voice and swollen, sore throat due to Wind-Heat?
A. Niu Bang Zi (Fructus Arctii)
B. Chan Tui (Periostracum Cicadae)
C. Sang Ye (Folium Mori)
D. Ju Hua (Flos Chrysanthemi)

5. Which of the following herbs can not only release Exterior but also treat childhood febrile diseases in which Wind causes convulsions, spasms, delirium, or night terrors?
A. Chan Tui (Periostracum Cicadae)
B. Sang Ye (Folium Mori)
C. Ju Hua (Flos Chrysanthemi)
D. Man Jing Zi (Fructus Viticis)

6. Which of the following herbs should be contraindicated in cases of pregnancy and for people who want to become pregnant because it can reduce sperm count and deform the fetus?

A. Sang Ye (Folium Mori)
B. Ju Hua (Flos Chrysanthemi)
C. Chan Tui (Periostracum Cicadae)
D. Man Jing Zi (Fructus Viticis)

7. Which of the following are actions of Sang Ye (Folium Mori Albae)?
A. Releases Exterior and expels Wind Heat, Expel Wind Damp and relieves pain, Stops internal Wind
B. Releases Exterior and expels Wind Cold, Relieves back pain from Wind Cold invasion
C. Expels Wind and clears Lung Heat, Clears Liver and brightens the eyes, Cool Blood and stops bleeding
D. Releases Exterior and expels Cold, warms the middle and stops vomiting, expels Cold and stops cough, regulates Ying and Wei

8. Which of the following are actions of Ju Hua (Flos Chrysanthemi Morifolii)?
A. Releases Exterior and expels Wind Heat, Expel Wind Damp and relieves pain, stops internal Wind
B. Releases Exterior and expels Wind Cold, relieves back pain from Wind Cold invasion
C. Expels Wind and clears Lung Heat, clears Liver and brightens the eyes, cool Blood and stops bleeding
D. Disperses Wind and clears Heat, clears Liver and brightens the eyes, calms the Liver and extinguishes Wind

9. Which of the following herbs can disperse Liver channel Wind-Heat manifesting as excessive tearing, red, painful, or swollen eyes, or floater in front of the eyes?
A. Man Jing Zi (Fructus Viticis)
B. Dan Dou Chi (Semen Sojae Praeparatum)
C. Fu Ping (Herba Spirodelae)
D. Mu Zei (Herba Equiseti Hiemalis)

10. Which of the following herbs can eliminate irritability and can be used for restlessness, stifling sensation in the chest and insomnia following febrile disorder?
A. Man Jing Zi (Fructus Viticis)
B. Dan Dou Chi (Semen Sojae Praeparatum)
C. Fu Ping (Herba Spirodelae)

D. Mu Zei (Herba Equiseti Hiemalis)

11. Which of the following herbs should be contraindicated for nursing mothers?
A. Man Jing Zi (Fructus Viticis)
B. Fu Ping (Herba Spirodelae)
C. Dan Dou Chi (Semen Sojae Praeparatum)
D. Mu Zei (Herba Equiseti Hiemalis)

12. Which of the following herbs can induce sweating and disperse Wind-Heat, vent rashes, stop itching and promote urination?
A. Fu Ping (Herba Spirodelae)
B. Mu Zei (Herba Equiseti Hiemalis)
C. Ge Gen (Radix Puerariae)
D. Chai Hu (Radix Bupleuri)

13. Which of the following herbs can be used for Wind-Heat affecting the eyes and causing redness, pain, swelling, cloudiness, blurred vision, pterygium, or excessive tearing and is used also as an auxiliary herb for Blood in the stool or hemorrhoids?
A. Fu Ping (Herba Spirodelae)
B. Mu Zei (Herba Equiseti Hiemalis)
C. Ge Gen (Radix Puerariae)
D. Chai Hu (Radix Bupleuri)

14. Which of the following herbs can be used for Exterior disorders lodged in the muscles manifesting in fever, headache, and stiff or tight upper back and neck?
A. Mu Zei (Herba Equiseti Hiemalis)
B. Ge Gen (Radix Puerariae)
C. Chai Hu (Radix Bupleuri)
D. Sheng Ma (Rhizoma Cimicifugae)

15. Which of the following herbs can stop thirst due to Stomach Heat, especially appropriate in cases of externally-contracted Heat and hasten recovery from measles with incomplete expression of the rash?
A. Mu Zei (Herba Equiseti Hiemalis)
B. Ge Gen (Radix Puerariae)
C. Chai Hu (Radix Bupleuri)
D. Sheng Ma (Rhizoma Cimicifugae)

16. Which of following herbs can raise the Yang to stop diarrhea and lower Blood pressure?
A. Mu Zei (Herba Equiseti Hiemalis)
B. Ge Gen (Radix Puerariae)
C. Chai Hu (Radix Bupleuri)
D. Sheng Ma (Rhizoma Cimicifugae)

17. Which of the following are actions of Chai Hu (Radix Bupleuri)?
A. Releases Exterior and expels Wind Heat, Expel Wind Damp and relieves pain, stops internal Wind
B. Releases Exterior and expels Wind Cold, relieves back pain from Wind Cold invasion
C. Expels Wind and clears Lung Heat, clears Liver and brightens the eyes, cool Blood and stops bleeding
D. Harmonizes Shao Yang and reduces fever, smooths Liver Qi, raises the Yang Qi

18. Which of the following are actions of Sheng Ma (Rhizome Clmicifugae)?
A. Release Exterior and vents rashes, clears Heat and relieves toxicity, raise the Yang Qi
B. Releases Exterior and expels Wind Cold, relieves back pain from Wind Cold invasion
C. Expels Wind and clears Lung Heat, clears Liver and brightens the eyes, cool Blood and stops bleeding
D. Harmonizes Shao Yang and reduces fever, smooths Liver Qi, raises the Yang Qi

19. Which of the following herbs can vent rashes in the cool-pungent herbs?
A. Bo He, Niu Bang Zi, Chan Tui
B. Fu Ping, Ge Gen, Sheng Ma
C. Both of A and B
D. Only A

20. Which of the following herbs can raise the Yang to stop diarrhea?
A. Ge Gen (Radix Puerariae)
B. Chai Hu (Radix Bupleuri)
C. Sheng Ma (Rhizoma Cimicifugae)
D. All of them

Answer Keys: 1D. 2D. 3B. 4B. 5A. 6C. 7C. 8D. 9A. 10B. 11C. 12A. 13B. 14B. 15B. 16B. 17D. 18A. 19C. 20D

Chapter 2 Herbs that Clear Heat

Classification:

1. Herbs that drain Fire
2. Herbs that clear Liver Heat and brighten eyes
3. Herbs that cool Blood
4. Herbs that clear Deficiency Heat
5. Herbs that clear Heat and dry Dampness
6. Herbs that clear Heat and relieve toxicity

Section 1 Herbs that Drain Fire

1. Shi Gao (Gypsum Fibrous) 石膏
2. Han Shui Shi (Calcitum Sue Gypsum Rubrum) 寒水石
3. Zhi Mu (Rhizoma Anemarrhenae) 知母
4. Zhi Zi (Gardeniae Fructus) 栀子
5. Dan Zhu Ye (Herba Lophateri) 淡竹叶
6. Lu Gen (Rhizoma Phragmitis) 芦根
7. Tian Hua Fen (Radix Trichosanthis) 天花粉
8. Xiong Dan (Fel Ursi) 熊胆
9. Ya Zhi Cao (Commelinae Herba) 鸭跖草
10. Xi Gua Pi (Citrulli Fructus) 西瓜皮
11. Lian Zi Xin (Plumuia Nelumbinis) 莲子心

Name	Property	CN	Actions & Indications	Remarks
Shi Gao (Gypsum Fibrosum) 石膏 Gypsum	Sweet Very Cold	LU ST	1. **Clears Qi stage Heat:** for Qi stage Heat of the four levels of disease, or the Yang Ming channel stage of the six stages of disease manifested as **4 bigs**: (1) **"Big fever"** without chills, (2) **"Big thirst,"** (3) **"Big sweating,"** (4) flooding, **"Big pulse,"** and red tongue with yellow coating; used with Zhi Mu, Gan Cao (such as Bai Hu Tang).	DOSAGE 15-60g The main ingredient in it is (CaSO4.2H2O).

			2. **Clears Lung Heat:** for cough and wheezing with fever due to Lung Heat; used with Ma Huang, Xing Ren, Gan Cao (such as Ma Xin Shi Gan Tang) 3. **Clears Stomach Heat:** for toothache, swollen and painful gums due to Stomach Fire; used with Huang Lian, Sheng Ma, Sheng Di Huang as in Qing Wei San. 4. **Promotes tissue regeneration:** topically use after being calcined for eczema, burns, and ulcerated sores.	
Han Shui Shi (Calcitum Sue Gypsum Rubrum) 寒水石 Calcitum	Acrid Cold Salty	HT ST KI	1. **Clears Heat:** for high fever, irritability, and thirst from Heat in the Qi stage, especially useful for warm pathogen diseases that occur during the summer. 2. **Drains Fire:** applied topically for burns and such problems as sore throat and oral ulcers.	l0-15g It is used instead of Shi Gao when it is not available.
Zhi Mu (Rhizoma Anemarrhenae) 知母 Anemarrhena rhizome	Bitter Cold	LU ST KI	1. **Clears Heat:** for Qi stage Heat manifested as high fever, irritability, bleeding gums, thirst; used with Shi Gao, Gan Cao (such as Bai Hu Tang). 2. **Stops cough:** for cough due to Lung Heat or Lung Yin Deficiency; used with Bei Mu (such as Er Mu San). 3. **Generates fluid:** for diabetes (wasting and thirsting disorder); used with Tian Hua Fen, Mai Men Dong. 4. **Nourishes Yin:** for steaming bone syndrome, irritability, afternoon fever, five centers Heat; or	6-12g

			spermatorrhea, nocturnal emissions, and abnormally elevated sex drive due to Yin Deficiency; used with Huang Bai, Sheng Di Huang, Shan Yao (such as Zhi Bai Di Huang Wan)	
Zhi Zi (Gardeniae Fructus) 栀子 Cape jasmine fruit Gardenia	Bitter Cold	HT LR	1. **Clears Heat and eliminates irritability:** for fever, irritability, restlessness, stifling sensation in the chest, insomnia, or delirious speech; used with Dan Dou Chi or Huang Lian, Huang Qin. 2. **Clears Damp-Heat:** for painful urinary dribbling (Lin syndrome), red eyes, or sores due to Damp-Heat; used with Mu Tong, Che Qiao Zi; For jaundice, used with Yin Chen, Da Huang (such as Yin Chen Hao Tang). 3. **Cools Blood and stops bleeding:** for nasal bleeding, vomiting Blood, or Blood in the stool or urine due to Blood Heat, after being charred; used with Sheng Di Huang, Mu Dan Pi. 4. **Resolves toxicity** for boils and sores due to Heat toxicity. Can be used orally or topically.	3-10g
Dan Zhu Ye (Herba Lophateri) 淡竹叶 Lophatherum stem and leaves	Sweet Bland Cold	HT SI ST	1. **Clears Heat and eliminates irritability:** for irritability and thirst due to Heat; used with Shi Gao, Zhi Zi. 2. **Promotes urination and clears Damp-Heat:** for scanty and painful urination (Lin syndrome), mouth sores and swollen, painful gums with irritability and a dark-red tip on the tongue due to Heat in the	10-15g

			Small Intestine channel; used with Sheng Di Huang, Mu Tong, Gan Cao (as inDao Chi San).	
Lu Gen (Phragmitis Rhizoma) 芦根 Reed Rhizomet	Sweet Cold	LU ST	1. **Clears Heat and generates Fluid:** for fever, irritability, and thirst due to Heat; used with Tian Hua Fen, Shi Gao. 2. **Clears Lung Heat:** for Lung abscess due to Lung Heat; used with Yin Hua, Pu Gong Yin. 3. **Stops vomiting:** for vomiting due to Stomach Heat; used with Zhu Ru, Huang Lian. 4. **Vents rash:** for febrile diseases with rashes that are incompletely expressed. 5. **Promotes urination:** for dark, scanty urine or Blood in the urine; used with Xiao Ji, Mu Tong.	**15-30g** Double dosage when fresh Lu Gen used. Wei Jing (stem of Lu Gen).
Tian Hua Fen (Trichosanthis Radix) 天花粉 Trichosanthis root Snake gourd root	Bitter Slightly Sweet Sweet Cold	LU ST	1. **Clears Heat and generates fluid:** for thirst and irritability due to Heat injured fluid, thirst from Yin Deficiency, and diabetes (wasting and thirst disorder); used with Ge Gen, Sheng Di Huang. 2. **Clears Lung Heat:** for cough with yellow Phlegm, thick-dry sputum or Blood-streaked sputum due to Lung Heat; used with Bei Mu, Sang Bai Pi, Jie Geng. 3. **Resolves toxicity and expels pus:** for hot toxic carbuncles and sores, breast abscess; used with Jin Yin Hua.	10-15g Do not use it for women who are pregnant or want to become pregnant.
Xiong Dan (Fel Ursi) 熊胆	Bitter, Cold	LV GB HT	1. **Extinguishes Wind and stop convulsion:** for convulsions due to Liver Heat. 2. **Clears Heat toxicity:** for carbuncles and	1-2g

Bear Gallbladder with dry bile			hemorrhoid. 3. **Clears Liver and brightens eyes:** for red, swollen, and painful eyes due to Liver channel Heat or Wind-Heat, photosensitivity, night blindness, and loss of vision	
Ya Zhi Cao (Commelinae Herba) 鸭跖草 Dayflower	Sweet, Bland, Cold	LU ST SI	1. **Clears Heat and drains Fire:** for the fever of relatively superficial Warm pathogen diseases. While this herb does have some toxicity-resolving action, it is rather weak. 2. **Clears Heat and promotes urination:** for hot painful urinary dribbling with urinary dysfunction and edema.	15-30g
Xi Gua Pi (Citrulli Fructus) 西瓜皮 Watermelon peel	Sweet, Cold	BL HT ST	1. **Clears Summer Heat and generates Fluids:** for Summer Heat patterns, especially those with significant thirst and dark, scanty urine and dry heaves.	15-30g
Lian Zi Xin (Nelumbinis Plumula) 莲子心 Lotus Plumule	Bitter Cold	HT PC	1. **Clear Heart Fire:** for warm-Heat pathogen diseases where Heat collapses into the Pericardium channel, causing mental confusion or delirium. Also for insomnia or irritability due to excessive Heart Fire. 2. **Stops bleeding:** for vomiting of Blood. 3. **Binds Essence:** for spermathorrhea.	1.5-3g

Practice 4

1. What is the function of Zhi Mu (Anemarrhenae rhizome)?
A. Clear Heat, purge Fire
B. Nourish Yin
C. Lubricate Dryness
D. All of the above

2. What is the common function of Shi Gao (Gypsum Fibrosum) and Zhi Mu (Anemarrhenae rhizome)?
A. Moisten Intestines
B. Clear deficient Heat
C. Nourish Yin and generate fluids
D. Clear Heat and purge Fire

3. Which herb do you choose in order to clear Heat, resolve irritability, cool the Blood and stop bleeding?
A. Shi Gao (Gypsum Fibrosum)
B. Zhi Mu (Anemarrhenae rhizome)
C. Lu Gen (Phragmitis rhizome)
D. Zhi Zi (Gardeniae Fructus)

4. Which herb is best for a patient who has fever, irritability, thirst and dysuria?
A. Shi Gao (Gypsum Fibrosum)
B. Zhi Mu (Anemarrhenae rhizome)
C. Lu Gen (Phragmitis rhizome)
D. Dan Zhu Ye (Laphatheri Herba)

5. Which herb can clear Heat reduce swelling, dispel pus, and generate body fluids?
A. Tian Hua Fen (Trichosanthis Radix)
B. Zhi Mu (Anemarrhenae rhizome)
C. Lu Gen (Phragmitis rhizome)
D. Dan Zhu Ye (Laphatheri Herba)

6. What are characters of Heat in Qi level?
A. Fever, slight aversion to Cold and Wind, reddish tongue tip, whitish thin or slightly yellow tongue coating, floating and rapid pulse, usually accompanied by headache, cough, dry mouth, slight thirst, and swelling pain of the throat.

B. Fever, aversion not to Cold but to Heat, vexation and thirst, sweating, reddish urine, reddish tongue, yellowish tongue coating, and rapid pulse.
C. Severe fever in the night, mild thirst, vexation and insomnia, or even delirium, appearance of macules and eruption, deep-red tongue with scanty coating, and thin and rapid pulse.
D. Worsened fever at night, restlessness, or even delirium, mania, appearance of purplish or blackish macules and eruptions, or hematemesis, epistaxis, hematochezia, hematuria, deep-red tongue, and rapid pulse.

7. Which of the following herbs can be used for toothache due to Stomach Fire and topically for eczema, burns, and ulcerated sores?
A. Shi Gao (Gypsum Fibrosum)
B. Zhi Mu (Anemarrhenae rhizome)
C. Lu Gen (Phragmitis rhizome)
D. Dan Zhu Ye (Laphatheri herba)

8. Which of the following herbs can be used for both Lung Heat and Lung Yin Deficiency coughing and bleeding gums?
A. Shi Gao (Gypsum Fibrosum)
B. Zhi Mu (Anemarrhenae rhizome)
C. Lu Gen (Phragmitis rhizome)
D. Dan Zhu Ye (Laphatheri Herba)

9. Which of the following herbs can be used for wasting and thirsting disorder (Diabetes)?
A. Zhi Mu (Anemarrhenae Rhizome)
B. Lu Gen (Phragmitis Rhizome)
C. Tian Hua Fen (Trichosanthis Radix)
D. All of above

10. Which of the following herbs can be used for insomnia or irritability due to excessive Heart Fire?
A. Shi Gao (Gypsum Fibrosum)
B. Lian Zi Xin (Lotus Plumule)
C. Lu Gen (Phragmitis Rhizome)
D. Dan Zhu Ye (Laphatheri Herba)

11. Which of the following herbs can be used for Summer Heat patterns, especially those with significant thirst and dark, scanty urine and dry heaves?
A. Xi Gua Pi (Watermelon Peel)

B. Lian Zi Xin (Lotus Plumule)
C. Lu Gen (Phragmitis Rhizome)
D. Dan Zhu Ye (Laphatheri Herba)

12. Which of the following herbs can promote urination?
A. Lu Gen (Phragmitis rhizome), Lian Zi Xin (Lotus Plumule)
B. Lu Gen (Phragmitis rhizome), Ya Zhi Cao (Dayflower)
C. Dan Zhu Ye (Laphatheri Herba), Tian Hua Fen (Trichosanthis Radix)
D. Xi Gua Pi (Watermelon Peel), Zhi Zi (Gardeniae Fructus)

13. Which of the following herbs can be used for steaming bone disorder, irritability, afternoon or low-grade fevers, Heat in the five centers, also for spermatorrhea, nocturnal emissions, and abnormally elevated sex drive?
A. Zhi Zi (Gardeniae Fructus)
B. Xi Gua Pi (Watermelon Peel)
C. Lu Gen (Phragmitis Rhizome)
D. Zhi Mu (Anemarrhenae Rhizome)

14. Which of the following herbs is good for Heat in the Blood with such as symptoms as nosebleed, vomiting Blood, or Blood in the stool or urine?
A. Zhi Zi (Gardeniae Fructus)
B. Lu Gen (Phragmitis Rhizome)
C. Tian Hua Fen (Trichosanthis Radix)
D. Lian Zi Xin (Lotus Plumule)

15. Which of the following herbs is good for Heat in the Small Intestine channel with the above symptoms plus irritability and a dark-red tip on the tongue?
A. Dan Zhu Ye (Laphatheri Herba)
B. Lu Gen (Phragmitis Rhizome)
C. Tian Hua Fen (Trichosanthis Radix)
D. Lian Zi Xin (Lotus Plumule)

16. Which of the following herbs is good for red, swollen, and painful eyes due to Heat or Wind-Heat in the Liver channel?
A. Dan Zhu Ye (Laphatheri Herba)
B. Lu Gen (Phragmitis Rhizome)
C. Xiong Dan (Bear Gallbladder)
D. Lian Zi Xin (Lotus Plumule)

17. Which paired herbs are common to use for Lung Abscess?
A. Lu Gen (Phragmitis Rhizome), Lian Zi Xin (Lotus Plumule)
B. Lu Gen (Phragmitis Rhizome), Tian Hua Fen (Trichosanthis Radix)
C. Dan Zhu Ye (Laphatheri Herba), Tian Hua Fen (Trichosanthis Radix)
D. Xi Gua Pi (Watermelon Peel), Zhi Zi (Gardeniae Fructus)

18. Which paired herbs are common to use for Heat in the Qi level?
A. Shi Gao (Gypsum Fibrosum), Zhi Mu (Anemarrhenae Rhizome)
B. Lu Gen (Phragmitis Rhizome), Tian Hua Fen (Trichosanthis Radix)
C. Dan Zhu Ye (Laphatheri Herba), Tian Hua Fen (Trichosanthis Radix)
D. Xi Gua Pi (Watermelon Peel), Zhi Zi (Gardeniae Fructus)

Answer Keys: 1D. 2D. 3D. 4D. 5A. 6B. 7A. 8B. 9D. 10B. 11A. 12B. 13D. 14A. 15A. 16C. 17B. 18A

Section 2 Herbs that Clear Liver Heat and Brighten Eyes

1. Xia Ku Cao (Spica Prunellae) 夏枯草
2. Jue Ming Zi (Semen Cassiae) 决明子
3. Qing Xiang Zi (Semen Celosiae) 青葙子
4. Mi Meng Hua (Flos Buddlejae) 密蒙花
5. Gu Jing Cao (Flos Eriocauli) 谷精草
6. Ye Ming Sha(Vespertilionis Faeces) 夜明砂

Name	Property	CN	Actions & Indications	Remarks
Xia Ku Cao (Spica Prunellae) 夏枯草 Selfheal spike, Prunella.	Bitter Acrid Cold	GB LR	1. **Clears Liver Fire and brightens eyes:** for red, painful, or swollen eyes due to Liver Fire upward-blazing, eye pain that increases in the evening due to Liver Deficiency; used with Ju Hua, Shi Jue Ming. 2. **Disperses nodules:** for any neck lump or nodule, such as scrofula, lipoma, swollen glands or goiter due to Phlegm-Fire. Also used for similar nodules in the inguinal canal and other parts of the body; used with Xuan Shen, Mu Li. 3. **Reduces Blood pressure:** for hypertension, especially when Liver Yang rising or with Liver Fire.	10-15g
Jue Ming Zi (Semen Cassiae) 决明子 Foetid cassia seeds	Bitter Sweet Cool	LR KI LI	1. **Clears Liver and brightens eyes:** for red, swollen, and painful eyes due to Heat or Wind-Heat in the Liver channel, photosensitivity, night blindness, and loss of vision. A) Liver Heat; used with Xia Ku	10-15g

			Cao B) Wind Heat, Used with Ju Hua, Gu Jing Cao. 2. **Subdues Liver Yang:** for headache and dizziness from ascending Liver Yang. Recently used for treating hypertension; used with Bai Shao, Gou Teng. 3. **Moistens Intestine:** for dry stools or chronic constipation; used with Dan Zhu Ye, Gua Lou Ren, Dang Gui. 4. **Prevents atherosclerosis:** for high cholesterol. It can lower both Blood pressure and serum cholesterol.	
Qing Xiang Zi (Semen Celosiae) 青葙子 Celosia seeds	Sweet Cool	LR	1. **Clears Liver, brightens the eyes:** for Wind-Heat or Liver Fire causing red, painful, swollen eyes, superficial visual obstruction, or cataract. A. For red, painful and swollen eyes or superficial visual obstruction; used with Ju Hua, Jue Ming Zi B. Hypertension due to ascendant Liver Yang; used with Ju Hua, Jue Ming Zi, Gou Teng.	6-15g **Wrapped** for decoction. It can induce dilatation of the pupils and may affect eye pressure. It is therefore contraindi-cated in patients with dilated pupils or elevated eye pressure, as in glaucoma.
Mi Meng Hua (Flos Buddlejae) 密蒙花 Buddleia flower	Sweet Cool	LR	**Clears Liver, brightens the eyes:** for red, swollen, painful eyes, excessive tearing, superficial visual obstruction, or sensitivity to light. Can be used	6-10g

bud			for either excess or Deficiency.	
Gu Jing Cao (Flos Eriocauli) 谷精草 Pipewort Scapus, Inflorescence	Sweet, Neutral	LR ST	1. **Disperses Wind-Heat, brightens the eyes:** for Wind-Heat entering the Liver channel causing red, swollen eyes, spots in front of the eyes, photosensitivity, excessive tearing, or pterygium. 2. **Also used for Wind-Heat:** headache, toothache, or throat painful obstruction.	6-15g
Ye Ming Sha (Vespertilionis Faeces) 夜明砂 Bat feces	Acrid, Cold	LR	1. **Clears the Liver and brightens the eyes:** for night blindness, superficial visual obstruction, and cataracts. 2. **Disperses Blood stasis and reduces accumulations:** for traumatic injury and accumulations from childhood nutritional impairment (Gan Ji).	6-15g Decocted in water for an oral dose. Wrapped for decoction. Contraindicated in patients with dilated pupils or elevated eye pressure, as in glaucoma.

Practice 5

1. Xia Ku Cao (Prunella or Selfheal spike) clears Liver Fire and
A. Eliminates Dampness
B. Moistens Dryness
C. Cools Blood
D. Disperses nodulation

2. Which herb can lower Blood pressure?
A. Tian Hua Fen (Trichosanthis Radix)
B. Jue Ming Zi (Cassiae Semen)
C. Lu Gen (Phragmitis Rhizome)
D. Dan Zhu Ye (Laphatheri Herba)

3. Which herb is good at red, swollen, and painful eyes due to Heat or Wind-Heat in the Liver channel and also for eye problems such as photosensitivity, night blindness, and loss of vision without visible physical changes to the eye?
A. Shui Niu Jiao (Bubali Cornu)
B. Sheng Di Huang (Rehmanniae Radix)
C. Mu Dan Pi (Moutan Cortex)
D. Jue Ming Zi (Cassiae Semen)

4. Which herbs can induce dilatation of the pupils and may affect eye pressure and therefore, contraindicated in patients with dilated pupils or elevated eye pressure, as in glaucoma?
A. Qing Xiang Zi (Semen Celosiae)
B. Ye Ming Sha (Vespertilionis Faeces)
C. Only A
D. Both of them

5. Which herbs need to be wrapped for decoction?
A.Qing Xiang Zi (Semen Celosiae)
B. Ye Ming Sha (Vespertilionis Faeces)
C. Only A
D. Both of them

6. Jue Ming Zi (Cassiae Semen) clears Liver, brightens eyes and
A. Moistens Intestine
B. Prevents atherosclerosis
C. Subdues Liver Yang
D. All of them

Answer Keys: 1D. 2B. 3D. 4D. 5D. 6D.

Section 3 Herbs that Clear Damp-Heat

1. The herbs in this category are primarily used for patterns of Damp-Heat such as dysenteric disorders, urinary difficulty or pain, jaundice, furuncles, and eczema.

2. Clinically, they are often combined with those that drain Fire or clear Heat and resolve toxicity.

3. Because of their Cold nature, they should not be used in cases of Spleen or Stomach Deficiency.

Herbs

1. Huang Qin (Radix Scutellariae) 黄芩
2. Huang Lian (Rhizoma Coptidis) 黄连
3. Huang Bai (Cortex Phellodendri) 黄柏
4. Ku Shen (Radix Sophorae Flavescentis) 苦参
5. Long Dan Cao (Radix Gentianae) 龙胆草
6. Qin Pi (Cortex Fraxini) 秦皮

Name	Property	CN	Actions & Indications	Remarks
Huang Qin (Radix Scutellariae) 黄芩 Baical Skullcap root, Scutellaria	Bitter Cold	GB LI LU ST	1. **Clears Damp-Heat:** for (1). diarrhea or dysentery due to Damp-Heat in the Stomach or Intestines; used with Huang Lian, Bai Shao, and Dang Gui (such as Shao Yao Tang). (2). Damp-Warmness with fever, stifling sensation in the chest, and thirst but with an inability to drink; Used with Huang Lian, Huang Bai, Zhi Zi. (3). Damp-Heat in the lower Jiao with painful urinary dribbling; used with Mu Tong, Hua Shi. (4). for Damp Heat jaundice as an auxiliary herb. 2. **Clears Lung Heat:** for cough with thick, yellow sputum. 3. **Clears Heat and resolves toxicity**:	3-10g Good for Upper Jiao

			for high fever/chills, irritability, and thirst, for sore throat, hot sores and swellings. 4. **Stops bleeding:** for internal excess Heat causing bleeding, including vomiting or coughing of Blood, nosebleed, and Blood in the stool; used with Sheng Di Huang. 5. **Calms fetus:** pacifies the womb when the fetus is restless or kicking excessively due to Heat; used with Dang Gui, Bai Shao.	
Huang Lian (Rhizoma Coptidis) 黄连 Coptis rhizome	Bitter Cold	HT LI ST LR	1. **Clears Damp Heat:** for (1). diarrhea or dysentery due to Damp-Heat in the Stomach or Intestines; used with Bai Shao, Dang Gui, Huang Qin (such as Shao Yao Tang) (2). vomiting and/or acid regurgitation due to Stomach Heat; used with Ban Xia, Huang Qin (such as Ban Xia Xie Xin Tang. 2. **Resolves Fire toxicity:** for (1). high fever, irritability, disorientation, delirium, red tongue, and a rapid and full pulse; used with Zhi Zi. (2). painful red eyes and sore throat, and for boils, carbuncles, and abscesses; used with Hung Qin, Huang Bai, Zhi Zi. 3. **Stops bleeding:** for nosebleed, or Blood in the urine, stool, or vomit due to Blood-Heat.	2-5g Good for Middle Jiao
Huang Bai (Cortex Phellodendri) 黄柏 Amur cork tree	Bitter Cold	KI BL	1. **Drains Damp-Heat:** for (1). Thick, yellow vaginal discharge, foul smelling diarrhea or dysentery; used with Qian Shi, Bai Guo (such as Yi Huang Tang) (2) red, swollen, and	5-10g Good for Lower Jiao

bark Phellodendron			painful knees, legs or feet due to Damp-Heat pouring downward; used with Bai Tou Weng, Qin Pi, Huang Lian (such as Bai Tou Weng Tang); Used with Cang Zhu (such as Er Miao San) (3). Damp-Heat jaundice; used with Zhi Zi (such as Zhi Zi Bai Pi Tang). 2. **Clears Deficiency Heat:** for steaming bone disorder, night sweats, afternoon fevers and sweating, sometimes accompanied by nocturnal emissions and spermatorrhea due to Kidney Fire ascending with Yin Deficiency; used with Shu Di Huang, Shan Yao, Mu Dan Pi (such as Zhi Bai Di Huang Wan). 3. **Resolves Fire toxicity:** for sores and Damp lesions of the skin due to Fire toxin; used with Huang Lian, Huang Qin.	
Ku Shen (Radix Sophorae Flavescentis) 苦参 Sophora root extract	Bitter Cold	BL HT LR LI SI	1. **Clears Damp Heat:** for Damp-Heat in the lower Jiao leading to jaundice, dysentery, vaginal discharge, and sores; used with Huang Bai, Huang Lian. 2. **Disperses Wind, kills parasites, and stops itching:** used both internally and topically for Damp toxin skin lesions manifestated as chronic itching, seepage, and bleeding. Also for genital itching and vaginal discharge; used with Che Qian Zi, Huang Bai. 3. **Promotes urination:** for painful urinary dribbling and hot edema	3-10g **Incompatible with Li Lu** (Veratri Nigri Radix et Rhizoma).

			due to Damp-Heat in the Small Intestine; used with Dan Zhu Ye, Mu Tong.	
Long Dan Cao (Radix Gentianae) 龙胆草 Chinese gentian root, Gentiana	Bitter Cold	GB LR ST	1. **Clears Liver and gallbladder Damp-Heat:** for (1). Red, swollen, sore throat and eyes, swollen and painful ears, or sudden deafness due to Damp-Heat in the upper part of the gallbladder channel; used with Zhi Zi, Che Qian Zi, Huang Qin (such as Long Dan Xie Gan Tang) (2). Damp-Heat in the Liver or Gallbladder channels (especially the lower parts) with jaundice, pain, swelling, or Dampness in the genital area, or foul-smelling vaginal discharge and itching; used with Yin Chen, Zhi Zi. 2. **Drains Liver Fire:** for headache or red eyes due to Liver Fire blazing upward; Liver Wind-Heat with fever, spasm, convulsion or flank pain; used with Huang Qin, Chai Hu, Zhi Zi, Ju Hua.	3-6g
Qin Pi (Cortex Fraxini) 秦皮 Korean ash branch bark	Bitter Cold	BL LR LI GB	1. **Clears Damp Heat, resolves toxicity:** for diarrhea, dysenteric disorder and vaginal discharge due to Damp-Heat; used with Bai Tou Weng, Huang Bai (such as Bai Tou Weng Tang). 2. **Clears Liver Fire and benefits eyes:** for Liver Heat affecting the eyes causing redness, swelling, pain, or the formation of superficial visual obstructions; used with Ju Hua, Long Dan Cao. 3. **Disperses Wind-Dampness:** for Bi syndrome, primarily of the hot type.	6-12g

			4. **Calms wheezing and stops cough:** for wheezing and cough due to Lung Heat.	

Practice 6

1. Which of following herbs is the best herb for Fire and Damp-Heat in the Liver and gallbladder?
A. Huang Lian (Rhizoma Coptidis)
B. Long Dan Cao (Radix Gentianae Longdancao)
C. Huang Qin (Radix Scutellariae Baicalensis)
D. Ku Shen (Sophora root)

2. Which of the following herbs is more effective for vaginal discharge and genital itching due to Damp-Heat in the lower jiao?
A. Huang Qin (Radix Scutellariae Baicalensis)
B. Ku Shen (Sophorae Flavescentis)
C. Long Dan Cao (Radix Gentianae Longdancao)
D. Da Qing Ye (Folium Daqingye)

3. What is the condition for using Long Dan Cao (gentianae radix)?
A. Diarrhea due to Spleen and Stomach Deficiency
B. Acid regurgitation due to Stomach Heat
C. Dysentery due to toxic Heat
D. Vaginal discharge and itching due to Damp-Heat

4. Which of the following herb can clear Lung Heat and Damp-Heat, stop bleeding as well?
A. Huang Qin (Radix Scutellariae Baicalensis)
B. Ku Shen (Sophorae Flavescentis)
C. Long Dan Cao (Radix Gentianae Longdancao)
D. Da Qing Ye (Folium Daqingye)

Answer Keys: 1B. 2B. 3D. 4A

Section 4 Herbs that Clear Heat and Resolve Toxicity

Common characteristics:

1. All of them are cool or Cold.
2. Most of them are bitter.
3. Most of them have antibiotic, antiviral, anti-inflammatory effects.

Cautions:

Contraindicated in diarrhea due to Spleen Deficiency.

Herbs:

1. Jin Yin Hua (Flos Lonicerae) 金银花
2. Ren Dong Teng (Caulis Lonicerae Japonicae) 忍冬藤
3. Lian Qiao (Fructus Forsythiae) 连翘
4. Da Qing Ye (Folium Isutidis) 大青叶
5. Ban Lan Gen (Radix Isatidis) 板蓝根
6. Yu Xing Cao (Herba Houttuyniae) 鱼腥草
7. Chuan Xin Lian (Andrographis paniculata (Burn. F.) Ness) 穿心莲
8. Qing Dai (Indigo naturalis) 青黛
9. Pu Gong Ying (Herba Taraxaci) 蒲公英
10. Zi Hua Di Ding (Herba Violae) 紫花地丁
11. Ye Ju Hua (Flos Chrysanthemi Indici) 野菊花
12. Zi Bei Tian Kui (herba begoniae) 紫背天葵
13. Bai Jiang Cao (Herba Patriniae) 败将草
14. Bai Hua She She Cao (Herba Hedyotidis Diffusae) 白花蛇舌草
15. Bai Tou Weng (Radix Pulsatillae) 白头翁
16. Ya Dan Zi (Bruceae Fructus) 鸭胆子
17. Ma Chi Xian (Herba Portulaceae) 马齿苋
18. Hong Teng (Caulis Sargentodoxae) 红藤
19. Bai Xian Pi (Cortex Dictamni) 白鲜皮
20. Ban Zhi Lian (Herba Scutellariae Barbatae) 半枝莲
21. Ban Bian Lian (Herba Lobeliae Chinensis) 半边莲
22. She Gan (Rhizoma Belamcandae) 射干
23. Ma Bo (Lasiophaera seu Calvatia) 马勃
24. San Dou Gen (Radix Sophorae Tonkinensis) 山豆根

25. Bei Dou Gen (Menispermi Rhizoma) 北豆根
26. Bai Guo (Semen Ginkgo) 白果
27. Shan Ci Gu (Cremastrae seu Pleiones Pseudobulbus) 山慈菇
28. Bai Lian (Ampelopsis Radix) 白蔹
29. Lou Lu (Radix Rhapontici seu Echinops) 漏芦
30. Lu Dou (Phaseoli radiati Semen) 绿豆
31. He Ye (Nelumbinis Folium) 荷叶
32. Pang Da Hai (Semen Sterculiae Lychnophorae) 胖大海
33. Chong Lou/Zao Xiu (Rhizoma Paridis) 重楼/蚤休
34. Wei Ling Cai (Potentillae chinensis Herba) 委陵菜
35. Tu Fu Ling (Rhizoma Smilacis Glabrae) 土茯苓
36. Chui Pen Cao (Sedi Herba) 垂盆草
37. Ji Xue Cao (Centellae Herba) 积雪草
38. Ji Gu Cao (Abri Herba) 鸡骨草
39. Tu Niu Xi (Radix Achyranthis) 土牛膝
40. Shi Shang Bai (Herba Selaginellae doederleinii) 石上柏
41. Long Kui (Solani nigri Herba) 龙葵
42. Wan Nian Qing (Rohdeae japonicae Radix et Rhizoma) 万年青

Name	Property	CN	Actions & Indications	Remarks
Jin Yin Hua (Flos Lonicerae) 金银花 Honeysuckle flower	Sweet Cold	LI LU ST	1. **Clears Heat and resolves Fire toxicity:** for hot, painful sores and swellings in various stages of development, especially of the breast, throat or eyes; used with Pu Gong Ying, Zi Hua Di Ding (such as Wu Wei Xiao Du Yin. Also for intestinal abscess, used with Lu Gen, Pu Gong Ying 2. **Expels Wind-Heat:** for the early stage of febrile diseases manifested as fever, slight sensitivity to Wind, sore throat, and headache; used with Lian Qiao, Dan Zhu Ye, Bo He, Niu Bang Zi (such as Yin Qiao San). Also for externally contracted Summer Heat.	10-15g

			3. Clears lower Jiao Damp-Heat: for Damp-Heat dysentery or Lin syndrome; used with Huang Bai, Che Qian Zi.	
Ren Dong Teng (Caulis Lonicerae Japonicae) 忍冬藤 Honeysuckle Stem	Sweet Cold	LI LU ST	**Similar as Jin Yin Hua** (Flos Lonicerae)	15-30g
Lian Qiao (Fructus Forsythiae) 连翘 Forsythia fruit	Bitter Slightly Acrid Cool	HT LR GB	1. **Clears Heat and resolves toxicity:** for external Wind-Heat with high fever, slight chills, sore throat, and headache; used with Jin Yin Hua, Pu Gong Ying. 2. **Reduces abscesses and dissipates clumps:** for external sores, internal abscesses, scrofula, or throat painful obstruction; used with Jin Yin Hua, Pu Gong Ying. 3. **Expels Wind-Heat:** for the early stage of febrile diseases with fever, slight sensitivity to Wind, sore throat, and headache; used with Jin Yin Hua, Dan Zhu Ye, Bo He, Niu Bang Zi (such as Yin Qiao San).	6-15g
Ban Lan Gen (Radix Isatidis) 板蓝根	Bitter Cold	HT ST	1. **Clears Heat, resolves Fire toxicity:** for febrile diseases, warm epidemic disorders, mumps; used with Lian Qiao, Niu Bang Zi, Huang Qi, Xuan Shen (such as Pu Ji Xiao Du Yin). 2. **Cools Blood and benefits throat:** for painful, swollen throat conditions and Damp-Heat jaundice; used with Niu Bang Zi, Jie Geng.	10-15g.

Da Qing Ye (Folium Isutidis) 大青叶 Woad leaf, Indigo	Bitter Very Cool	HT LU ST	1. **Clears Heat and resolves Fire toxicity:** for (1) hot, painful sores and swellings in various stages of development, especially of the breast, throat, or eyes; used with She Gan, Shan Dou Gen. Also for intestinal abscess. (2) Wind Heat or epidemic febrile outbreak; used with Jin Yin Hua, Pu Gong Ying. 2. **Cools Blood and dissipates maculae:** for maculae or other skin eruptions with fever, irritability, and changes of consciousness due to Heat in the Blood. Also used for vomiting of Blood; used with Xi Jiao, Sheng Di Huang.	10-15g
Yu Xing Cao (Herba Houttuyniae) 鱼腥草 Houttuynia	Acrid Cool	LI LU	1. **Clears Heat:** for Lung abscess or Lung Heat cough with expectoration of thick, yellowish green sputum. Also used both internally and topically for toxic sores. A. Cough due to Lung Heat or Lung abscess; used with Jin Yin Hua, Jie Geng, Lu Gen. B. Toxic sores; used with Lian Qiao, Pu Gong Ying external or internal. 2. **Drains Damp-Heat and promotes urination:** for diarrhea due to large Intestine Damp-Heat or painful urinary dribbling (Lin syndrome) due to Damp-Heat in the Lower Burner; used with Jin Qian Cao, Shi Wei, Bai Mao Gen.	15-30g Do not decoct longer.
Chuan Xin Lian	Bitter Cold	LI LU	1. **Clears Heat and resolves Fire toxicity:** for many kinds of Heat	6-10g

(Andrographis paniculata (Burn. F.) Ness) 穿心莲 Green chiretta		SI ST	disorders including Heat in the Lung Heat cough, sore throat and Lin syndrome. Also for Fire toxin manifestations on the skin such as sores and carbuncles; used with Jin Yin Hua; can be applied topically (fresh form of herb) for snakebites. 2. **Clears Damp-Heat and stops diarrhea:** for Damp Heat dysentery, hot painful urinary dribbling and eczema; used with Ma Chi Xian.	
Qing Dai (Indigo naturalis) 青黛 Natural indigo	Salty Cold	LR LU	1. **Clears Heat and resolves toxicity:** for hot, painful sores and swellings; used with Xi Jiao, Xuan Shen, Shi Gao. 2. **Cools the Blood, and reduces maculae:** for maculae or bleeding due to Blood Heat or other warm toxin; used with Sheng Di Huang, Mu Dan Pi. 3. **Drains Liver Fire and stops tremor**: for convulsions due to Liver Fire. 4. **Clears Liver Fire, cools Blood:** for cough and chest pain due to Liver Fire accosting the Lung.	**1.5-3g** Used in pill or powder form.
Pu Gong Ying (Herba Taraxaci) 蒲公英 Dandelion	Bitter Sweet Cold	LR ST	1. **Clears Heat and resolves toxicity:** for abscesses and sores, especially useful for breast and intestinal abscesses and particularly when they are firm and hard; used with Ju Hua, Xia Ku Cao, Huang Qin. Can be used both internally and topically. A) Breast abscess; used with Zhe	**10-30g**

			Bei Mu, Mo Yao. B) Lung abscess; used with Yu Xing Cao, Lu Gen. C) Large Intestine abscess; used with Chi Shao, Da Huang, Bai Jiang Cao. D) Sores; used with Jin Yin Hua, Zi Hua Di Ding. 2. **Clears Damp Heat:** for Damp-Heat jaundice and Lin syndrome (painful urinary dribbling); used with Yin Chen Hao. 3. **Clears throat and benefit the eyes:** for sore throat and redness and swelling eyes.	
Zi Hua Di Ding (Herba Violae) 紫花地丁 Yedeon's violet	Bitter Acrid Cold	HT LR	1. **Clears hot sores:** for sores and abscesses; used with Jin Yin Hua, Pu Gong Ying, Yie Ju Hua (as in Wu Wei Xiao Du Yin). 2. **Clears Heat and resolves toxicity:** for red, swollen eyes; swollen, painful throat and ears; mumps, and snakebite. A. Red, swollen eyes due to Liver Heat; used with Ju Hua, Chan Tui. B. For toxic snake bite, make juice and mix with Xiong Huang.	**15-30g**
Ye Ju Hua (Flos Chrysanthemi Indici) 野菊花 Wild Chrysanthemum flower	Bitter Acrid Slightly Cold	LU LR	1. **Clears Heat and resolves Fire toxicity:** for furuncles, carbuncles, sores, sore throat due to Fire toxicity and red eyes caused by Wind Heat. 2. Internal taking and external wash for itching due to Wind Dampness. A. Furuncles, carbuncles and sores; used with Jin Yin Hua, Pu	10-15g

			GongYing. B. Sore, swollen throat and red eyes due to Fire; used with Sang Ye, Xia Ku Cao.	
Zi Bei Tian Kui (Tian Kui Zi) (Herba Begoniae) 紫背天葵 Begonia			1. **Reduces swelling, and disperses clumping:** for abscesses, swelling, toxic sores, and deep-rooted furuncles. Recently used for some types of cancer.	9-15g
Bai Jiang Cao (Herba Patriniae) 败酱草 Patrinia, Thiaspi	Bitter Acrid Slightly Cold	LI LR ST	1. **Clears Heat toxicity, expels pus:** for internal intestinal, or Lung abscess, surface sores and swellings. Can be taken internally or applied topically. A) Intestinal abscess at early stage without pus; used with Jin Yin Hua, Mu Dan Pi. B) Intestinal abscess with pus; used with Yi Yi Ren, Fu Zi (such as Yi Yi Fu Zi Bai Jiang San C) Lung abscess; used with Yu Xing Cao, Lu Gen, and Jie Geng. D) Sores and carbuncles; used with Pu Gong Ying. 2. **Moves Blood and stops pain:** for abdominal and chest pain, postpartum pain, and post-operative pain due to Heat-induced Blood stasis; used with Wu Ling Zhi, Xiang Fu or use alone.	6-15g
Bai Hua She She Cao (Herba Hedyotidis	Bitter Sweet Cold	LR LI ST	1. **Clears Fire toxicity:** for intestinal abscess, toxic sores, ulcerations, and swellings. Also for snakebites. Recently, it is used	**15-30g**

Diffusae) 白花蛇舌草 Heydyotis, Oldenlandia			for cancers. A. Intestinal abscess; used with Bai Jiang Cao. B. Toxic sores ulcerations and swellings; used with Jin Yin Hua, Lian Qiao. C. Hot painful urinary dysfunction; used with Shi Wei, Bai Mao Gen. 2. **Clears Damp-Heat, promotes urination:** for hot painful urinary dribbling and Damp-Heat jaundice; used with Yin Chen Hao, Jin Qian Cao.	
Bai Tou Weng (Radix Pulsatillae) 白头翁 Chinese anemone root, Pulsatilla	Bitter Cold	LR LI ST	1. **Cools Blood and stops dysentery:** primarily for Bloody dysentery, amebic dysentery due to Damp-Heat in the Stomach or Intestines; used with Qin Pi, Huang Lian (such as Bai Tou Weng Tang). 2. **Clears Heat and resolves toxicity:** for mumps, scrofula, carbuncles, due to Fire toxicity; used with Pu Gong Ying, Lian Qiao.	6-15g
Ya Dan Zi Bruceae Fructus 鸭胆子 Java brucea fruit, Brucea	Bitter, Cold **Toxic**	LI LR	1. **Clears Heat and resolves toxicity:** for chronic or recurring dysentery especially chronic Cold stagnation dysentery (Xiu Xi Li) that wax and wane, or alternating hard and soft stools. It is also used for amebic dysentery. 2. **Checks malaria:** for malarial disorders. 3. **Used topically for warts and corns:** either as a paste or an ointment.	**0.5-2g** It should be put in capsules, or traditionally placed within fresh Long Yan Rou (Longan Arillus).

			4. **Treats cancers**, Recently used for cancers, specifically for colon or breast cancer.	
Ma Chi Xian (Herba Portulaceae) 马齿苋 Purslane, Portulaca	Sour Cold	LI LR	1. **Resolves Fire toxicity and cools Blood:** for dysentery due to Damp-Heat or Fire toxin. 2. **Clears Damp-Heat and treats sores:** for Fire toxin carbuncles or sores, and red-and-white vaginal discharge; used with Huang Qin, Huang Lian. 3. **Stops bleeding:** for uterine bleeding (especially postpartum), painful Bloody urinary dribbling, and hot painful urinary dribbling; used with Mu Tong, Xiao Ji. 4. Taken as an antidote for the pain and swelling of wasp stings and snakebite; used with Pu Gong Ying.	9-15g
Hong Teng (Caulis Sargentodoxae) 红藤 Sargentodoxa vine	Bitter Neutral	LI LR	1. **Clears Heat, resolves toxicity:** for intestinal abscess and skin lesions with Heat, swelling, and pain. 2. **Invigorates the Blood and disperses stasis:** for trauma, dysmenorrhea, and joint pain.	9-15g
Bai Xian Pi (Cortex Dictamni) 白鲜皮 Dictamnus root bark	Bitter Cold	SP ST	1. **Clears Heat toxicity, expels Wind, and dries Dampness:** for Wind-Heat or Damp-Heat sores, carbuncles and rashes leaking yellow fluid, or itching vaginal pruritis with discharge; used with Ku Shen, She Chuang Zi. 2. **Clears Damp-Heat:** for jaundice, used with Yin Chen Hao. For Bi syndrome, used with Cang Zhu,	6-10g

			Huang Bai.	
Ban Zhi Lian (Herba Scutellariae Barbatae) 半枝莲 Barbat Skullcap, Scutellaria	Acrid Bitter Cold	LI LR LU	1. **Clears Heat, resolves toxicity,:** for furuncles, sores, and abscesses, as well as snakebite and trauma. 2. **Promotes urination:** for edema or ascites of cirrhosis due to Damp-Heat. 3. **Stops bleeding:** for trauma, vomiting Blood, nosebleeds, or painful Bloody urinary dribbling.	**15-30g**
Ban Bian Lian (Herba Lobeliae Chinensis) 半边莲 Lobelia	Sweet Neutraul	HT LU SI	1. **Resolves toxicity:** for carbuncles, boils and tonsillitis due to Heat toxicity and snake bite. A. Poisonous snakebite, wasp stings and initial stage of carbuncles and sores; used with Huang Qin, Huang Lian, Jin Yin Hua. 2. **Promotes urination:** for edema with big abdomen; used with Ze Xie, Zhu Ling.	10-15g
She Gan (Rhizoma Belamcandae) 射干 Blackberry lily, Leopard flower	Bitter Cold	LU	1. **Clears Heat, resolves toxicity, benefits throat:** for swelling and pain of the throat due to Fire excess, Fire toxin, or Phlegm-Heat obstruction. Sometimes used alone for sore throat; used alone or with Huang Qin, Jie Geng. 2. **Transforms Phlegm and clears Lung:** for cough and wheezing with Phlegm obstruction; used with Xing Ren, Jie Geng.	3-10g
Ma Bo (Lasiophaera seu Calvatia) 马勃 Fruiting Body of Puffball,	Acrid Neutral	LU	1. **Clears Lung, resolves Fire toxicity, and benefits the throat:** for Fire toxin affecting throat causing pain, swelling, and loss of voice and cough due to Lung Heat; used with Ban Lan Gen, Xuan	1.5-5g **wrapped** in cheesecloth

Lasiosphaera			Shen. 2. **Stops bleeding:** used both internally and topically to stop bleeding of oral cavity lips and gums.	
Shan Dou Gen (Radix Sophorae Tonkinensis) 山豆根 Subprostrate, Sophora root	Bitter Cold	LI LU	1. **Clears Heat toxicity and benefits throat:** for swollen, painful throat, both internally and as a gargle; used with Niu Bang Zi and Jie Geng. 2. **Clears Heat toxicity and reduces swelling:** for abscess and toxic sores. Now it is used for cancer, especially of throat and Lung cancer; used with Xing Ren.	3-6g
Bei Dou Gen (Menispermi Rhizoma) 北豆根 Asiatic moonseed rhizome	Bitter Cold	LU ST LI	1. **Clears Heat and resolves toxicity:** for sore throat, cough, and mumps due to Wind Heat affecting the Lungs and Stomach . 2. **Dispels Wind and stops pain:** for Wind-Damp painful obstruction.	3-9g
Shan Ci Gu (Cremastrae seu Pleiones Pseudobulbus) 山慈菇 Indian iphigenia bulb	Sweet Slightly Acrid Cold	LR ST	1. **Clears Heats, resolve toxicity, reduces abscesses, and dissipates nodules:** for sores, abscesses, carbuncles, scrofula, and Phlegm nodules. 2. **Resolves toxicity, dissipates nodules, and reduces swellings:** recently used for masses, primarily in the abdomen, including those due to tumors.	3-6g
Bai Lian Ampelopsis Radix 白蔹 Ampelopsis, Japanese ampelopsis root	Bitter, Acrid, Neutral Cold	HT ST LV	1. **Clears Heat, resolves toxicity, reduces abscesses, disperses clumps, and generates flesh:** for clogging collections of Heat toxin leading to sores and abscesses.	3-10g Incompatib-le with Radix Aconiti **(Wu Tou).**
Lou Lu (Radix	Bitter Salty	LI ST	1. **Clears Heat, resolves toxicity, and reduces sores and swellings:** for the	5-9g

Rhapontici seu Echinops) 漏芦 Common swisscentaury root	Cold		early stages of sores and abscesses when they are red, swollen, and painful. 2. **Promotes lactation:** for insufficient lactation, especially when there are signs of Heat.	
Lu Dou (Phaseoli radiati Semen) 绿豆 Mung bean	Sweet Cold	HT ST	1. **Clears Summer Heat:** for irritability and fever, due to Summer Heat. It is often made as a soup in the summer time to prevent Summer Heat. 2. **Clears Heat and resolves toxicity:** for toxic sores and swellings. 3. **Antidote:** as an antidote for poisoning due to Zhi Fu Zi (Aconiti Radix lateralis preparata) or fava beans.	15-30g
He Ye (Nelumbinis Folium) 荷叶 Lotus leaf	Bitter, Slightly Sweet, Neutral	HT SP LR	1. **Clears Summer Heat:** for fever, irritability, excessive sweating, scanty urine, and diarrhea due to Summer Heat; used with Lu Dou, Bai Bian Dou. 2. **Raises Spleen Yang:** for diarrhea due to Spleen Deficiency; used with Bai Zhu, Bai Bian Dou 3. **Stops bleeding:** for bleeding in the lower Jiao due to Heat or stagnation; used with Ce Bai Ye, fresh Ai Ye, Shen Di (as Si Sheng Wan).	3-10g
Pang Da Hai (Semen Sterculiae Lychnophorae) 胖大海 Boat Sterculia Seed	Sweet Cold	LU LI	1. **Clears Heat, nourishes Lung and benefits throat:** for sore throat, loss of voice; used with Jie Geng, Niu Bang Zi. 2. **Clears Heat and moves the bowel:** for constipation with headache, red eyes, toothache; used with Jie Geng, Chan Tui, Bo He.	2-4 pieces. Dunked with boiled water.

Practice 7

1. Common function of Xia Ku Cao (Prunellae Spica) and Long Dan Cao (Gentianae Radix)?
A. Clear HT
B. Clear LU
C. Clear LV
D. Clear ST

2. Which of the following herbs is very commonly used for intestinal abscess?
A. Pu Gong Ying (Dandelion)
B. Ban Lan Gen (Woat root or Isatis root)
C. Bai Jiang Cao (Patrinia or Thiaspi)
D. Yu Xing Cao (Houtuynia)

3. Which of the following herbs is very commonly used for Lung abscess?
A. Ju Hua (Flos chrysanthemi morifolii)
B. Ban Lan Gen (woat root or Isatis root)
C. Bai Jiang Cao (Patrinia or Thiaspi)
D. Yu Xing Cao (Houtuynia)

4. Which of the following herbs is very commonly used for breast abscess?
A. Pu Gong Ying (Dandelion)
B. Ban Lan Gen (Woat root or Isatis root)
C. Bai Jiang Cao (Patrinia or Thiaspi)
D. Yu Xing Cao (Houtuynia)

5. Which of the following satements is the function of Shan Dou Gen (Radix Sophorae Tonkinensis)?
A. Relieve Exterior Wind-Cold and clear Heat
B. Clear Heat and dry the Dampness
C. Clear Heat, resolve Fire toxicity and benefit throat
D. Clear Heat, relieve toxicity and invigorate the Blood

6. Which of the following herbs has the functions of clearing Heat and relieving Fire toxicity, expelling external Wind-Heat and clearing Damp-Heat from the lower-Jiao, and is the one of the best for skin sores, carbuncles and epidemic febrile diseases at Wei level?
A. Jin Yin Hua (Honeysuckle flower or Lonicera)

B. Da Qing Ye (Folium Daqingye)
C. Pu Gong Ying (Herba Taraxaci Mongolici cum Radice)
D. Bai Jiang Cao (Patrinia or Thiaspi)

7. Ban Lan Gen (Radix Isatidis seu Baphicacanthi) is one of the best herb for ___________.
A. Sore and swollen throat due to toxic Heat
B. Skin sores, carbuncles and internal abscesses
C. The Heat in the Ying and Blood level during the epidemic febrile disease
D. Dysentery due to Damp-Heat

8. Da Qing Ye (Folium Daqingye) is one of the best herbs for which of the following?
A. Sore and swollen throat due to toxic Heat
B. Skin sores, carbuncles and internal abscesses
C. Heat in the Ying level and early Blood level during epidemic febrile disease
D. Dysentery due to Damp-Heat

9. Ye Ju Hua (Flos Chrysanthemi Indici) has the function of which of the following?
A. Clearing deficient Heat
B. Clearing Heat and relieving toxicity
C. Clearing Heat and cooling the Blood
D. Purging downward

10. Chuan Xin Lian (Andrographis paniculata (Burn. F.) Ness) is the best herb for which of the following?
A. Breast abscess
B. Lung abscess
C. Dysentery due to Damp-Heat or Fire toxin
D. Cough, sore throat due to Lung-Heat

11. Which of the following herb has all the following functions: clearing Heat and relieving toxicity, expelling external Wind-Heat and dissipating nodules?
A. Jin Yin Hua (Flos Lonicerae Japonicae)
B. Lian Qiao (Fructus Forsythiae Suspensae)
C. Da Qing Ye (Folium Daqing ye)
D. Ban Lan Gen (Radix Isatidis seu Baphicacanthi)

12. Which of following herb is an important herb for chronic Cold stagnation dysenteric disorders (Xiu Xi Li) that wax and wane, or alternating hard and soft stools?

A. Bai Tou Weng (anemone)
B. Ya Dan Zi (Bruceae Fructus)
C. Ma Chi Xian (Portulaca)
D. Hong Teng (Sargentodoxa vine)

13. Which of the following herb can resolve Fire toxicity, cool the Blood, clear Damp-Heat, stop bleeding and unblock painful urinary dribbling and is also used as an antidote for the pain and swelling of wasp stings and snakebite?
A. Bai Xian Pi (Cortex of Chinese dittany root)
B. Ban Zhi Lian (Herba Scutellariae Barbatae)
C. Ban Bian Lian (Lobelia)
D. Ma Chi Xian (Portulaca)

14. Which of the following herb can not only be used for Intestinal abscess and skin lesions with Heat, swelling, and pain but also for trauma, dysmenorrhea, and joint pain?
A. Ban Bian Lian (Lobelia)
B. Ban Zhi Lian (Herba Scutellariae Barbatae)
C. Hong Teng (Sargentodoxa vine)
D. She Gan (Belamcanda Rhizome)

15. Which of the following herb can clear Damp-Heat to stop itching and is used for vaginal pruritis with discharge?
A. She Gan (Belamcanda Rhizome)
B. Ma Bo (Lasiosphaera)
C. Shan Dou Gen (Sophora root)
D. Bai Xian Pi (Cortex of Chinese Dittany root)

16. What is the common action between Ban Zhi Lian (Herba Scutellariae Barbatae) and Ban Bian Lian (Lobelia)?
A. Clear Heat and resolve toxicity
B. Promote urination and reduce edema
C. Both A and B
D. Only A

17. Which herb does not benefit the throat?
A. She Gan (Belamcanda Rhizome)
B. Ban Lan Gen (Woat root or Isatis root)
C. Shan Dou Gen (Sophora root)

D. Yu Xing Cao (Houtuynia)

18. Which of the following statements is correct?
A. She Gan (Belamcanda Rhizome) can transform Phlegm and clear the Lungs, while Ma Bo (Lasiosphaera) can stop bleeding.
B. Ma Bo (Lasiosphaera) should be wrapped in cheesecloth, and decocted in water for an oral dose.
C. Both can clear Heat, resolve toxicity and improve the condition of throat.
D. All of them.

19. Which of the following herb is not toxic?
A. Ya Dan Zi (Bruceae Fructus)
B. Bai Guo (Semen Ginkgo)
C. Lu Dou (Mung Bean or phaseolus)
D. Xi Xin(Asarum)

20. Which of the following herb can astringe Lung, stop wheezing, stop excessive vaginal discharge and stabilize essence and control urination?
A. Bai Guo (Semen Ginkgo)
B. Bai Lian (Ampelopsis Radix)
C. Lu Dou (Mung bean or Phaseolus)
D. Ya Dan Zi (Bruceae Fructus)

21. Which of the following herb can clear Heat, resolve toxicity, reduce abscesses, disperse clumps, and generate flesh?
A. Bai Guo (Semen Ginkgo)
B. Bai Lian (Ampelopsis Radix)
C. Lu Dou (Mung bean or Phaseolus)
D. Ya Dan Zi (Bruceae Fructus)

22. Which of the following herb is often made as a tea in the summertime to prevent the occurrence of summer-Heat?
A. Bai Guo (Semen Ginkgo)
B. Bai Lian (Ampelopsis Radix)
C. Lu Dou (Mung Bean or phaseolus)
D. She Gan (Belamcanda Rhizome)

Answer Keys: 1C. 2C. 3D. 4A. 5C. 6A. 7A. 8C. 9B. 10C. 11B. 12B. 13D. 14C. 15D. 16C. 17D. 18D. 19C. 20A. 21B. 22C

Section 5 Herbs that Cool Blood

1. All of them can be used for Heat entering the Nutritive and Blood level of febrile diseases marked by a red tongue, irritability, restlessness, changes in consciousness and bleeding.

2. Herbs in this group clear Heat and Nourish Yin. The Cold property also makes them treat Yin Deficiency Heat.

Herbs:

1. Xi Jiao (Cornu Rhinoceri) 犀角
2. Shui Niu Jiao (Bubali Cornu) 水牛角
3. Sheng Di Huang (Radix Rehmanniae) 生地黄
4. Xuan Shen (Radix Scrophulariae) 玄参
5. Mu Dan Pi (Cortex Moutan Radicis) 牡丹皮
6. Chi Shao (Radix Paeoniae Rubra) 赤芍
7. Zi Cao (Radix Arnebiae) 紫草

Name	Property	CN	Actions & Indications	Remarks
Xi Jiao (Cornu Rhinoceri) 犀角 Rhinoceros horn	Bitter Salty Cold	HT LR ST	1. **Clears Heat and cools Blood:** for febrile diseases at Xue (Blood) level with bleeding; used with Shao Yao, Mu Dan Pi (as in Xi Jiao Di Huang Tang); Epidemic febrile diseases at Ying (Nutritive) level with high fever, unconsciousness and delirium; used with Sheng Di, Mu Dan Pi (Qing Yin Tang). 2. **Clears Heat and stops tremor:** for high fever, spasm and convulsion due to Heat entering the Heart and Liver during febrile disease; used with Ling Yang Jiao.	1.5-3g Can not be used with **Wu Tou** (including Chuan Wu and Cao Wu).
Shui Niu Jiao (Bubali Cornu)	Salty Cold	HT LR ST	1. **Clears Heat and cools Blood:** for high fever with bleeding due to febrile diseases affecting the	15-30g in decoction; 6-15g as a

水牛角 Water Buffalo Horn			Nutritive or Blood levels. 2. **Resolves Fire toxicity:** for sores and abscesses.	powder.
Sheng Di Huang (Radix Rehmanniae) 生地黄 Rehmannia, Chinese foxglove root	Sweet Bitter Cold	HT LR KI	1. **Clears Heat and cools Blood:** for high fever, thirst, and a scarlet tongue of febrile diseases due to Heat entered the Nutritive or Blood level. A. Epidemic febrile diseases at Xue (Blood) level; used with Shao Yao, Mu Dan Pi (such as Xi Jiao Di Huang). B. Epidemic febrile diseases at Ying (Nutritive) level with high fever, unconsciousness and delirium; used with Sheng Di Huang , Mu Da Pi (such as Qing Ying Tang). C. Febrile disease at late stage with lingering low-grade fever; used with Qing Hao, Bie Jia. D. Mouth and tongue sores or irritability, insomnia due to Heart Fire flaming up; used with Mu Tong, Gan Cao, Dan Zhu Ye (such as Dao Chi San). 2. **Nourishes Yin and generates fluid:** for dry mouth, continuous low-grade fever and constipation due to Yin Deficiency with injury of fluid, sore throat associated with Yin Deficiency and wasting and thirst disorder (Xiao Ke, diabetes); used with Mai Men Dong, Sha Shen, Ge Gen, Tian Hua Fen.	10-15g
Xuan Shen (Radix Scrophulariae) 玄参	Bitter Sweet Salty Cold	KI LU ST	1. **Clears Heat and cools Blood:** for Heat that has entered Blood level of febrile diseases with bleeding, fever, dry mouth, and a purplish	10-15g Antagonistic with **Li Lu** (Veratri Nigri

Ningpo figwort root, Scrophularia			tongue; used with Shi Gao, Xi Jiao, Zhi Mu. **2. Nourishes Yin:** for sore throat, constipation and irritability due to the warm-Heat pathogen diseases at the Ying level; used with Sheng Di Huang, Xi Jiao **3. Clears Heat and resolves toxicity:** for red eyes due to Liver Heat, sore throat due to Heat-toxicity. **4. Softens hardness and dissipates nodules:** for neck lumps due to Phlegm-Fire and severe throat pain and swelling. A. Sore throat or swollen and red eyes; used with Jie Geng, Niu Bang Zi B. Neck lumps due to Phlegm-Fire; used with Mu Li, Bei Mu.	Radix et Rhizoma).
Mu Dan Pi (Cortex Moutan Radicis) 牡丹皮 Tree peony root cortex	Acrid Bitter Cool	HT LR KI	**1. Clears Heat and cools Blood:** for (1). nose bleeding, Blood in the sputum or vomit, or subcutaneous bleeding when Heat entering the Blood level of warm-Heat pathogen disease with. (2). frequent and profuse menstruation due to Heat in the Blood; used with Shi Gao, Xi Jiao, Zhi Mu. **2. Clears Deficiency Heat:** for steaming bone disorder due to Yin Deficiency; used with Qing Hao, Bie Jia (as Qing Hao Jie Jia Tang). **3. Moves Blood:** for amenorrhea, dysmenorrhea, abdominal masses, lumps, or bruises due to traumatic injury due to Liver Blood stasis; used with Tao Ren , Gui Zhi, Fu	6-12g

			Ling (as Gui Zhi Fu Ling Wan). **4. Drains pus and reduces swelling:** for firm, non-draining sores and intestinal abscess. A) For Intestinal abscess, used with Da Huang, Tao Ren (as Da Huang Mu Dan Tang). B) For sores, used with Jin Yin Hua, Lian Qiao.	
Chi Shao (Radix Paeoniae Rubra) 赤芍 Red peony root	Sour Bitter Slightly Cold	LR SP	**1. Clears Heat and cools Blood:** for causing bleeding, fever, dry mouth, and a purplish tongue due to Heat entered Blood level of febrile diseases. **2. Moves Blood and stops pain:** for dysmenorrhea, amenorrhea, abdominal mass, stroke and injury. **3. Clears Liver Fire:** for red, swollen, and painful eyes, superficial visual obstruction.	6-12g **Antagonistic with Li Lu** (Veratri Nigri Radix et Rhizoma).
Zi Cao (Radix Arnebiae) 紫草 Groomwell root, Lithospermum	Sweet Cold	HT LR	**1. Cools the Blood and vents rashes:** for measles or chickenpox which are not progressing well; used with Lian Qiao. **2. Resolves Fire toxicity:** topically used for carbuncles, Damp-Heat skin lesions, burns or vaginal itching; used with Huang Bai.	5-10g

Practice 8

1. Which herb can clear Blood-Heat, Nourish Yin and generate body fluids?
A. Sheng Di Huang (Rehmanniae Radix)
B. Shui Niu Jiao(Bubali Cornu)
C. Mu Dan Pi(Moutan Cortex)
D. Zi Cao (Arnebiae Radix)

2. Which herb can activate Blood, remove stasis, and also clear deficient Heat?
A. Sheng Di Huang (Rehmanniae Radix)
B. Shui Niu Jiao (Bubali Cornu)
C. Mu Dan Pi (Moutan Cortex)
D. Zi Cao (Arnebiae Radix)

3. What herb is best for a patient who is suffering from severe Heat-toxin, with an inability of dark-purple rashes to erupt?
A. Shui Niu Jiao (Bubali Cornu)
B. Sheng Di Huang (Rehmanniae Radix)
C. Mu Dan Pi (Moutan Cortex)
D. Zi Cao (Arnebiae Radix)

4. What are the indications of Xuan Shen (scrophulariae radix)?
A. Swollen, painful, dry throat
B. Lump or lipoma due to Phlegm Fire
C. Warm disease, Heat in the Blood causing purpura
D. All of the above

5. Which herb can clear Heat to cool Blood and clear Heat to arrest tremor?
A. Xi Jiao (Cornu Rhinoceri)
B. Shui Niu Jiao (Bubali Cornu)
C. Sheng Di Huang (Radix Rehmanniae)
D. Xuan Shen (Radix scrophulariae)

6. Which of the following herbs is incompatible with Wu Tou (Radix Aconiti Carmichaeli)?
A. Xi Jiao (Cornu Rhinoceri)
B. Shui Niu Jiao (Bubali Cornu)
C. Sheng Di Huang (Radix Rehmanniae)

D. Xuan Shen (Radix scrophulariae)

7. Which of the following herbs is incompatible with Li Lu (Radix et Rhizoma Veratri)?
A. Xi Jiao (Cornu Rhinoceri)
B. Shui Niu Jiao (Bubali Cornu)
C. Sheng Di Huang (Radix Rehmanniae)
D. Xuan Shen (Radix Scrophulariae)

8. Which of the following herbs can clear Heat and cool Blood, move Blood, stop pain, clear Liver Fire as well?
A. Shui Niu Jiao (Bubali Cornu)
B. Sheng Di Huang (Radix Rehmanniae)
C. Xuan Shen (Radix scrophulariae)
D. Chi Shao (Radix Paeoniae Rubra)

9. Which of the following herbs can be used for a patient with constipation, irritability, sore throat, bleeding, fever, dry mouth, and a purplish tongue due to the epidemic febrile diseases at the Ying level?
A. Sheng Di Huang (Radix Rehmanniae), Xuan Shen (Radix Scrophulariae), Xi Jiao (Cornu Rhinoceri)
B. Shi Gao (Gypsum fibrous), Zhi Mu (Rhizoma Anemarrhenae), Zhi Zi (Gardeniae Fructus)
C. Bo He (Herba Menthae), Niu Bang Zi (Fructus Arctii), Sang Ye (Folium Mori)
D. Xia Ku Cao (Spica Prunellae), Jue Ming Zi (Semen Cassiae), Qing Xiang Zi (Semen Celosiae)

Answer Keys: 1A. 2C. 3D. 4D. 5A. 6A. 7D. 8D. 9A

Section 6 Herbs that Clear Deficient Heat

1. Qing Hao (Herba Artemisiae Annuae) 青蒿
2. Di Gu Pi (Cortex Lycci Radicis) 地骨皮
3. Bai Wei (Radix Cynanchi Atrati) 白薇
4. Yin Chai Hu (Radix Stellariae) 银柴胡
5. Hu Huang Lian (Picrorhizae Rhizoma) 胡黄连

Name	Property	CN	Actions & Indications	Remarks
Qing Hao (Herba Artemisiae Annuae) 青蒿	Bitter Cold	KI LR GB	1. **Checks malaria:** for alternative fever and chills of malaria. It is one of the best antimalarial medicine among western and Chinese Herbal Medicine; used fresh alone, or used with Huang Qin, Zhu Ru, (as in Hao Qin Qing Dan Tang). **2. Clears Deficiency Heat:** for fever as sequelae of febrile diseases; used with Bie Jia, Mu Dan Pi, Shen Di Huang as in Qing Hao Bie Jia Tang. **3. Cools Blood:** for Yin Deficiency Heat manifested as fever worse at night and better in the morning; used with Sheng Di Huang, Mu Dan Pi, Ce Bai Ye. **4. Clears Summer Heat:** for Summer Heat with low fever, headache, dizziness, and a stifling sensation in the chest; used with Lu Dou, He Ye.	6-12g. Do not decoct longer.
Di Gu Pi (Cortex Lycci Radicis) 地骨皮	Sweet Cold	LU LR KI	**1. Clears Heat and reduces steaming:** for night sweats, steaming bone disorder with sweating, chronic low-grade fever, irritability, and thirst due to Kidney and Liver Yin Deficiency; used with Zhi Mu, Bie Jia. **2. Cools the Blood and stops bleeding:** for febrile diseases with bleeding, such	**6-15g**

			as purpuric rashes or nosebleed due to Heat in the Blood; used with Ce Bai Ye, Bai Mao Gen. 3. **Clears Lung Heat:** for Lung Heat cough or wheezing; used with Sang Bai Pi, Gan Cao, Jing Mi (such as Xie Bai San).	
Bai Wei (Radix Cynanchi Atrati) 白薇	Bitter Salty Cold	LU ST KI	1. **Clears Heat and cools Blood:** for Yin deficient fever, postpartum fever, and lingering fever after febrile disease that injures the Blood or Yin; used with Sheng Di, Xuan Shen. 2. **Promotes urination and stops bleeding:** for hot or painful Bloody urinary dribbling (Bloody Lin), especially before or after giving birth; used with Mu Tong, Hua Shi, Shi Wei. 3. **Resolves toxicity:** for toxic sores, swollen and painful throat, and snake bite. 4. **Nourishes Yin:** for Exterior syndrome with Yin Deficiency; used with Yu Zhu as in Jia Jian Wei Rui Tang.	3-12g
Yin Chai Hu (Radix Stellariae) 银柴胡	Sweet Cool	LR ST	1. **Clears Deficiency Heat:** for steaming bone disorder due to Yin Deficiency Fire, or Yin deficient fever; used with Qing Hao, Di Gu Pi, Hu Huang Lian (such as Qing Gu San). 2. **Clears Heat and reduces childhood nutritional impairment:** for fever, thirst, and irritability associated with childhood nutritional impairment (Gan Ji) due to accumulation with Heat; used with Huang Qi, Hu Huang Lian.	3-9g
Hu Huang Lian (Picrorhizae Rhizoma)	Bitter Cold	LR ST LI	1. **Clears Deficiency Heat:** for steaming bone disorder due to Yin Deficiency . 2. **Clears Heat and reduces childhood nutritional impairment:** for abdominal	1.5-9g

胡黄连			distention, afternoon fevers, and dysenteric diarrhea associated with childhood nutritional impairment (Gan Ji). 3. **Drains Damp-Heat:** for Damp-Heat dysentery or sores.	

Practice 9

1. Which "clearing deficient Heat" herb can clear Summer Heat and stop malaria?
A. Qing Hao (Herba Artemisiae Annuae)
B. Di Gu Pi (Cortex Lycci Radicis)
C. Bai Wei (Radix Cynanchi Atrati)
D. Yin Chai Hu (Radix Stellariae)

2. Which of the following herb can cool Blood, reduce Bone-steaming emission of Heat, and Clear and Drain Lung Heat?
A. Hu Huang Lian (Picrorhizae Rhizoma)
B. Zhi Mu (Anemarrenha rhizome)
C. Di Gu Pi (Cortex ofwolfberry root/lycium bark)
D. Huang Bai (Phellodendron)

3. Which "clearing deficient Heat" herb can cool the Blood, promote urination and resolve toxicity?
A. Qing Hao (Herba Artemisiae Annuae)
B. Ban Bian Lian (Herba Lobeliae Chinensis)
C. Bai Wei (Radix Cynanchi Atrati)
D. Yin Chai Hu (Radix Stellariae)

4. Which of the following herbs can treat childhood nutritional impairment manifested by fever, thirst, and irritability due to Heat?
A. Hu Huang Lian (Picrorhizae Rhizoma), Qing Hao (Herba Artemisiae Annuae)
B. Yin Chai Hu (Radix Stellariae), Di Gu Pi (Cortex ofwolfberry root/lycium bark)
C. Qing Hao (Herba Artemisiae Annuae), Di Gu Pi (cortex ofwolfberry root/lycium bark)
D. Hu Huang Lian (Picrorhizae Rhizoma), Yin Chai Hu (Radix Stellariae)

5. Which of the following herb is the best one for steaming bone due to Kidney Fire with Deficiency Heat manifested as night sweats, steaming bone disorder with sweating, chronic low grade fever, irritability, and thirst?
A. Qing Hao (Herba Artemisiae Annuae)
B. Di Gu Pi (Cortex Lycci Radicis)
C. Bai Wei (Radix Cynanchi Atrati)
D. Yin Chai Hu (Radix Stellariae)

Answer Keys: 1A. 2C. 3C. 4D. 5B

Chapter 3 Purgative Herbs

Classification:

1. Purgatives
2. Mild purgatives
3. Drastic Purgatives

Main Indication:

Constipation due to accumulation of Cold or Heat.

Contraindication:

Exterior and Deficiency syndromes
The elderly
Pregnancy, postpartum during menstruation, and nursing mothers.
SP and ST Deficiency

Section 1 Purgatives

1. Da Huang (Radix et Rhizoma Rhei) 大黄
2. Mang Xiao (Mirabilitum) 芒硝
3. Fan Xie Ye (Folium Sennae) 番泻叶
4. Lu Hui (Herba Aloes) 芦荟

Name	Property	CN	Actions & Indications	Remarks
Da Huang (Radix et Rhizoma Rhei) 大黄 Rhubarb	Bitter Cold	LI HT LR	1. **Drains Heat and purges accumulations:** for high fever, profuse sweating, thirst, constipation, abdominal distention and pain, intestinal abscess; used with Mang Xiao, Zhi Shi, Hou Po (as in Da Cheng Qi Tang). **2. Clears Heat and drains Fire:** for sore throat, hot, swollen, and painful eyes, Fire toxin sores due to Heat or burn, Used with Jin Yin Hua, Pu	5-10g, **decoct it near the end.** It is called the 'general'. Alcohol prepared is good for moving Blood.

			Gong Ying, Lian Qiao for sores; used with Mu Dan Pi, Mang Xiao, Tao Ren for intestinal abscess. 3. **Clears Damp-Heat and promotes urination:** for edema, jaundice, painful urinary dribbling (Lin syndrome), hot type dysentery due to Damp-Heat; used with Yin Chen Hao, Zhi Zi, or with Mu Tong, Che Qian Zi. 4. **Cools Blood:** for Blood in the stool, vomiting Blood or nosebleed accompanied by constipation; used with herbs that clear Heat to stop bleeding. 5. **Moves Blood:** for amenorrhea, fixed abdominal masses, fixed pain due to Blood stasis, or traumatic injury or Intestinal abscess; used with Tao Ren, Hong Hua, Dang Gui.	Charred is good for stopping bleeding.
Mang Xiao (Mirabilitum) 芒硝 Mirabilite	Bitter Acrid Salty Cold	LI ST	1. **Purges accumulation and softens hardness:** for abdominal pain with constipation due to Heat in the Stomach and Intestines; used with Da Huang, Hou Po, Zhi Shi as in Da Cheng Qi Tang. 2. **Clears Heat and reduces swelling:** for red, swollen, painful eyes; painful, swollen, ulcerated mouth or throat; and red, swollen skin lesions, early stage of breast abscess; used with Peng Sha, Bing Pian.	10-15g Dissolved in warm water. **Incompatible with Liu Huang**. Topically use to stop lactation.
Fan Xie Ye (Folium Sennae) 番泻叶 "Imported purgative	Sweet Bitter Cold	LI	1. **Drains downward and guides out stagnation:** for constipation due to Heat accumulation in the Intestines. Can be used for both acute and chronic problems; used along or with Zhi Shi, Hou Po. Usually taken	**1.5-3g** taken alone as tea. 2-6g as decoction. Added near the end. Side

leaves" Senna leaf			alone as tea.	effects include nausea, vomiting, abdominal pain.
Lu Hui (Herba Aloes) 芦荟 Aloe	Bitter Cold	LI LR ST	1. **Drains Fire** for constipation, dizziness, red eyes, and irritability due to Heat accumulation; used with Long Dan Cao, Zhi Zi, Qing Dai 2. **Clears Liver Heat:** for epigastric discomfort, dizziness, headache, tinnitus, irritability, constipation due to Heat in Liver channel; used with Long Dan Cao, Huang Qin. 3. **Kills parasites:** for childhood nutritional impairment (Gan Ji), especially when it is related to roundworm. Also used for tinea; used with Shan Yao, Nan Gua Zi.	**1-2g**. Used in pills or capsules; do not decoct. Contraindicat-ed in pregnancy.

Section 2 Mild Purgatives

Main indication:

Constipation due to Blood, Yin, or Qi Deficiency.

Herbs:

1. Huo Ma Ren (Fructus Cannabis) 火麻仁
2. Yu Li Ren (Semen Pruni) 郁李仁

Name	Property	CN	Actions & Indications	Remarks
Huo Ma Ren (Fructus Cannabis) 火麻仁 Marijuana	Sweet Neutral	**LI** SP ST	1. **Moistens Intestine:** for elderly constipation, constipation after febrile disease, postpartum constipation due to Blood Deficiency. A. Constipation in the elderly; used with Dang Gui, Shu Di Huang, Xin Ren B. Yin Deficiency with constipation, or habitual constipation; used with Da Huang , Hou Po, Bai Shao (such as Ma Zi Ren Wan). C. Sores and ulcerations, oral or topical application.	10-15g; crush before decocting.
Yu Li Ren (Semen Pruni) 郁李仁 Bush Cherry pit	Sweet Neutral Bitter Acrid	**LI** SI SP	**1. Moistens Intestines:** for constipation due to Qi Deficiency or Yin and Blood Deficiency; used with Huo Ma Ren, Bai Zi Ren, Xing Ren as in Wu Ren Wan. **2. Promotes urination and reduces edema:** for edema with urinary difficulty; used with Sang Bai Pi, Chi Xiao Dou, Bai Mao Gen.	6-12g; crush before decocting.

Section 3 Drastic Purgatives

Main indication:

Constipation with stagnation of fluid in the thoracic or abdominal cavities.

Common characteristics:

1. Drive out water anally and forcefully for hydrothorax, ascites or edema.
2. Toxic
3. Contraindicated for pregnancy and Deficiency syndromes.
4. Low dosage given
5. Some can be used externally for abscess or carbuncle
6. Only for excessive syndrome

Herbs

1. Gan Sui (Radix Kansui) 甘遂
2. Da Ji (Radix Euphorbiae Pekinensis) 大戟
3. Yuan Hua (Flos Genkwa) 芫花
4. Shang Lu (Radix Phytolaccae) 商陆
5. Qian Niu Zi (Semen Pharbitidis) 牵牛子
6. Ba Dou (Semen CrotonTiglii) 巴豆

Name	Property	CN	Actions & Indications	Remarks
Gan Sui (Radix Kansui) 甘遂 Kan sui root	Bitter Cold **Toxic**	**LI** KI LU	1. **Drives out water and thin mucus:** for severe fluid retention in the chest and abdomen, general edema, and abdominal distention; used with Da Ji, Yuan Hua, Da Zao (such as Shi Zao Tang). 2. **Drives out Phlegm:** for seizures due to Wind-Phlegm or withdrawal mania due to Phlegm. 3. **Clears Heat and reduces swelling:** used topically for swollen, painful, nodular skin lesions due to Damp-Heat.	**0.5-1.5g** 1. **Only for excessive syndrome** **2. Incompatible with Gan Cao.** Side effects include nausea, vomiting, palpitations, abdominal pain, backache and

				hematuria.
Jing Da Ji (Radix Euphorbiae Pekinensis) 大戟 Peking spurge root, euphorbia	Bitter Cold **Toxic**	**LI** KI LU	1. **Drives out water and thin mucus:** for severe fluid retention in the chest and abdomen, general edema, and abdominal distention; used with Gan Sui, Yuan Hua (such as Shi Zao Tang). 2. **Reduces swelling and dissipates nodules:** used topically for red, swollen, painful, toxic sores or scrofula.	**1.5-3g** **Incompatible with Gan cao.** It is similar as Gan Sui but weaker.
Yuan Hua (Flos Genkwa) 芫花 Genkwa flower	Bitter Acrid Warm **Toxic**	**LI** KI LU	1. **Drives out water and thin mucus:** for accumulation of fluids in the chest and abdomen and thin mucus in the flanks; used with Gan Sui, Da Ji, Da Zao (such as Shi Zao Tang) 2. **Dispels Phlegm and stops cough:** for coughing and wheezing due to Phlegm. 3. **Kills parasites:** used topically for tinea.	**1.5-3g** **Incompatible with Gan Cao**
Shang Lu (Radix Phytolaccae) 商陆 Poke root, phytolacca	Bitter Cold **Toxic**	UB KI **LI** SP	1. **Drives out water and promotes urination:** for edema associated with constipation and urinary difficulty; used with Fu Ling, Bing Lang, Chi Xiao Dou, or use alone 2. **Reduces sores and carbuncle:** the fresh herb is used topically for hot-type sores. The fresh herb is commonly used.	5-10g. It is highly toxic. Use with great caution.
Qian Niu Zi (Semen Pharbitidis) 牵牛子 Morning glory seeds, pharbitis	Bitter Cold **Toxic**	**LI** KI LU	1. **Drives out water and promotes urination:** for general edema and ascites water retention or Dampness. 2. **Drives out Phlegm** for cough and wheezing, with sensation of fullness in the chest and abdomen due to thin mucus obstructing the Lungs; used with Ting Li Zi, Xing Ren, Hou Po	3-6g. Crush before decocting. **Incompatible with Ba Dou (Rotonis Fructus).**

			3. **Unblocks the bowels and removes accumulation:** for constipation due to Damp-Heat or food stagnation in the Stomach and Intestines. 4. **Expels Intestinal parasites**. For worms; used with Bing Lang as (such as Niu Lang Wan).	Can be toxic if it is used with large doses leading to hematuria and neurological disorders.
Ba Dou (Semen Croton Tiglii) 巴豆 Croton seed	Acrid Hot **Toxic**	ST KI LU	1. **Warmly unblocks and vigorously purges:** for constipation and abdominal fullness, distention, and pain due to Cold accumulation in the interior; used with Gan Jiang, Da Huang (such as San Wu Bei Ji Wan). 2. **Drives out water and reduces edema:** for ascites due to end-stage schistosomiasis; used with Xin Ren. 3. **Breaks up Phlegm and benefits throat:** for Phlegm clogging the throat leading to breathing difficulty, wheezing, severe fullness and distention in the chest and diaphragm. 4. **Promotes the healing of abscesses and ulcer:** used topically for suppurated abscesses which are not ulcerated, severe ulcers; used with Ru Xiang, Mo Yao.	**0.1-0.3g in pill** per day. **Incompatible with Qian Nu Zi.** At present a defatted preparation called Ba Dou Shuang (Crotonis Fructus Pulveratum) is used. Croton oil in it can cause diarrhea in doses as low as 0.01g. Twenty drops taken internally will be fatal because of massive fluid loss.

Practice 10

1. Which of the following statement about cathartic/laxative herbs is NOT correct?
A. They are classified by purgatives, mild purgatives and drastic purgatives.
B. Their main indication is constipation due to accumulation of Heat or Cold
C. They can purge large Intestine, drain Heat and discharge water retention.
D. They can be used in cases of Exterior syndrome.
E. They should stop taking the herb when the condition gets better

2. What is Da Huang's (Radix et Rhizoma Rhei) main indication?
A. Constipation due to Cold stagnation
B. Constipation due to post-partum Blood Deficiency
C. Constipation due to Yin Deficiency due to old age
D. Constipation due to Heat stagnation

3. If one wants to make use of Da Huang's purgative effect, how should it be cooked?
A. Decocted in advance
B. Decocted with the other herbs as usual
C. Decocted in filter
D. No more than 10 minutes (boiled later that means add near the end)

4. Which of the following herb has the following actions: 1. Drain Heat and purge accumulations; 2. drain Fire; 3. Clear Damp-Heat, and promote urination; 4. Drain Blood Heat; 5. Move Blood?
A. Da Huang (Radix et Rhizoma Rhei)
B. Mang Xiao (Mirabilitum)
C. Fan Xie Ye (Folium Sennae)
D. Lu Hui (Herba Aloes)

5. Which of the following statement about Da Huang (Radix et Rhizoma Rhei) is correct?
A. Contraindicated in cases of Exterior disorders; Contraindicated in cases of Qi or Blood Deficiency and Cold from Deficiency of the Spleen and Stomach
B. Caution during pregnancy, menstruation or post partum; Caution for nursing mothers
C. Alcohol prepared to move Blood; Charred to stop bleeding.
D. All of them

6. Which of the following herb is incompatible with Liu Huang?
A. Da Huang (Radix et Rhizoma Rhei)
B. Mang Xiao (Mirabilitum)
C. Fan Xie Ye (Folium Sennae)
D. Lu Hui (Herba Aloes)

7. Which of the following statement about Mang Xiao (Mirabilitum) is correct?
A. Contraindicated in cases of Spleen Deficiency and in the elderly.
B. Contraindicated during pregnancy, menstruation and post partum.
C. Topically used to stop lactation
D. All of them

8. Which of the following herb will cause abdominal pain, nauseas and vomiting if overdose and should be added near the end if decocted?
A. Da Huang (Radix et Rhizoma Rhei)
B. Mang Xiao (Mirabilitum)
C. Fan Xie Ye (Folium Sennae)
D. Lu Hui (Herba Aloes)

9. Which of the following herb can drain Fire and guide out accumulation, clear Liver Heat and kill parasites?
A. Da Huang (Radix et Rhizoma Rhei)
B. Mang Xiao (Mirabilitum)
C. Fan Xie Ye (Folium Sennae)
D. Lu Hui (Herba Aloes)

10. Which of the following statement about Huo Ma Ren (Fructus Cannabis) and Yu Li Ren (Semen Pruni) is NOT correct?
A. Both can moisten Intestine
B. Huo Ma Ren has sides effect if overdose or long term use; Yu Li Ren does not have any side effects.
C. Huo Ma Ren can promote urination and reduces edema; Yu Li Ren can not.
D. Both should be crushed before decoction.

11. Which of the following herbs can be used with Gan Cao?
A. Gan sui (Radix Kansui)
B. Da Ji (Radix Euphorbiae Pekinensis)
C. Yuan Hua (Flos Genkwa)
D. Shang Lu (Radix Phytolaccae)

12. Gan Sui (Radix Kansui) (Radix Euphorbiae Kansui), Da Ji (Radix Euphorbiae Pekinensis), and Yuan Hua (Flos Genkwa) all treat:
A. Traumatic injuries and pain
B. Wind Damp impediment conditions
C. Poisonous snake bites
D. Abdominal ascites and fluid accumulation in the chest and abdomen

13. Which of the following herbs is very hot and very poisonous?
A. Da Ji (Radix Euphorbiae Pekinensis) (Herba Euphorbiae Pekinensis)
B. Ba Dou (Semen Crotonis Tiglii)
C. Lu Hui (Herba Aloes)
D. Huo Ma Ren (Semen Cannabis Sativae)

Answer Keys: 1D. 2D. 3D. 4A. 5D. 6B. 7D. 8C. 9D. 10C. 11D. 12D. 13B

Chapter 4 Herbs that Promote Urine and Drain Dampness

1. **Actions:**
   ①. Promote urination
   ②. Treat Lin syndrome
   ③. Treat jaundice

2. **Indications:**
   ①. Edema
   ②. Urination retention
   ③. Lin syndrome
   ④. Jaundice
   ⑤. Damp carbuncle
   ⑥. Eczema
   ⑦. Diarrhea
   ⑧. Excessive vaginal discharge
   ⑨. Damp Bi syndrome
   ⑩. Phlegm retention

3. **Classification:**
   ①. Herbs that benefit urination for treating edema
   ②. Herbs that benefit urination and treat urinary tract disorder
   ③. Herbs that benefit urination and treat jaundice

4. **Caution and contraindications:**
   Yin Deficiency.

Section 1 Herbs that Benefit Urination for Treating Edema

Indications:

1. Edema (including renal edema, cardiac edema, hepatic edema)
2. Urination retention
3. Diarrhea

4. Phlegm retention

Herbs:

1. Fu Ling (Poria) 茯苓
2. Zhu Ling (Polyporus) 猪苓
3. Ze Xie (Rhizoma Alismatis) 泽泻
4. Yu Mi Xu (Stylus et Stigma Zeae Maydis) 玉米须
5. Yi Yi Ren (Semen Coicis) 薏苡仁
6. Chuan Mu Tong (Caulis Clematidis Armandii) 川木通
7. Chi Xiao Dou (Semen Phaseoli) 赤小豆
8. Dong Gua Pi (Exocarpium Benincaasae) 冬瓜皮

Name	Property	CN	Actions & Indications	Remarks
Fu Ling (Poria) 茯苓 Sclerotium of Tuckahoe, China-root, Poria, Boelen	Sweet Bland Neutral	HT SP LU	1. **Promotes urination:** for all kind of edema, urinary retention whether it is Cold, Heat, Deficiency or Excess syndrome. A) For Damp Heat syndrome; used with Mu Tong, Che Qian Zi B) For Damp Cold syndrome; used with Fu Zi, Gan Jiang. 2. **Tonifies Spleen:** for poor appetite, fatigue, loose stool and diarrhea due to Spleen Deficiency; used with Dang Shen, Bai Shu, and Gan Cao (such as Si Jun Zi Tang). 3. **Resolves Phlegm:** for dizziness, shortness of breath, cough, palpitation and vomiting due to Phlegm; used with Ban Xia, Chen Pi, Gan Cao (such as Er Chen Tang) 4. **Calms spirit (Shen):** for insomnia and palpitation due to Heart and Spleen Deficiency. A) Due to Deficiency of both Spleen and Heart; used with Dang Shen, Long Yan Rou, Suan Zao Ren B) Due to Phlegm retention in the	10-15g **Fu Ling Pi** 茯苓皮 (Peel of Fu Ling) is good for promoting urination. **Fu Shen** 茯神 (Poria cum Radix Pini, Fu Ling with tree root inside) is good for calming Shen.

			interior or due to disharmony between the Heart and Kidney; used with Yuan Zhi, Wu Wei Zi.	
Zhu Ling (Polyporus) 猪苓 Polyporus sclerotium	Sweet Bland Slightly cool	SP KI BL	**Promotes urination:** for 1. Edema, urinary retention; 2. Diarrhea due to Spleen Deficiency; 3. Lin syndrome and excessive vaginal discharge due to Heat, or Damp-Heat; 4. Jaundice due to Damp-Heat; used with Fu Ling, Ze Xie; Huang Bai, Che Qian Zi (such as Wu Ling San or Zhu Ling Tang).	5-10g
Ze Xie (Rhizoma Alismatis) 泽泻 Water Plantain, Rhizome, Alisma	Sweet Bland Cold	KI BL	**1. Promotes urination:** for edema, urinary retention, and diarrhea, dizziness due to water or Phlegm retention. **2. Clears lower Jiao Damp-Heat:** for Lin syndrome, excessive vaginal discharge due to lower Jiao Damp-Heat; used with Zhu Ling, Fu Ling (such as Wu Ling San). **3. Clears Kidney deficient Fire:** for night sweating, spermatorrhea, tinnitus, and lower back soreness due to Kidney Yin Deficiency (As in Liu Wei Di Huang Wan).	5-10g There are Alisol A and B in it.
Yu Mi Xu (Stylus et Stigma Zeae Maydis) 玉米须 Cornsilk	Sweet Neutral	BL G B LR	**1. Promotes urination:** for edema, urinary retention, Lin syndrome; used with Hai Jin Sha. **2. Clears Damp-Heat:** for both Yin and Yang type of jaundice; used with Yin Chen Hao, Jin Qian Cao. **3. Reduces BP:** for hypertension.	**30-60g**
Yi Yi Ren (Semen	Sweet Bland	SP ST	**1. Promotes urination:** for edema, urinary retention, abdominal	**10-30g**

Coicis) 薏苡仁 **(Yi Mi** 薏米) Seeds of Job's tears, coix	Slightly Cold	LU	distention due to Spleen Deficiency with water retention; used with Dong Gua Pi. **2. Tonifies Spleen:** for poor appetite and diarrhea due to Spleen Deficiency; used with Fu Ling, Chi Xiao Dou, Mu Tong. **3. Expels pus:** for Lung and intestinal abscess due to Lung Heat or intestinal Damp-Heat; used with Lu Gen, Dong Gua Ren, Tao Ren; Bai Jiang Cao, Mu Dan Pi. **4. Expels Wind Dampness:** for Bi syndrome, especially hot or Damp Bi syndrome; used with Ma Huang for Wind-Damp-Cold; used with Fang Ji, Sang Zhi for Wind-Damp-Heat.	
Chuan Mu Tong (Caulis Clematidis Armandii) 川木通 Akebia Caulis	Bitter cool	HT SI BL	**1. Promotes urination:** for edema, Lin syndrome, urinary retention, Damp Bi syndrome; used with Che Qian Zi, Ze Xie **2. Promotes lactation:** for insufficient lactation; used with Tong Cao, Wang Bu Liu Xing.	5-10g Another Mu Tong is called Guan Mu Tong 关木通 (Caulis Aristolochiae Manshuriensis) which is banned because of causing Chronic Renal Failure.
Chi Xiao Dou (Semen Phaseoli) 赤小豆 Aduki bean, phaseolus	Sweet Sour Neutral	HT SI	**1. Promotes urination:** for edema, urinary retention due to Kidney Deficiency. **2. Expels pus:** for abscess, carbuncles due to Damp-Heat. **3. Clears Damp-Heat:** for jaundice due to Dampness.	10-30g

Dong Gua Pi (Exocarpium Benincaasae) 冬瓜皮 Winter melon peel	Sweet Slightly Cold	LU SI	**1. Promotes urination:** for edema, especially Heat type, used with Fu Ling, Ze Xie. **2. Stops thirst:** for thirst due to Summer Heat, used with Chi Xiao Dou, He Ye.	**15-30g**

Practice 11

1. Which of the following herbs can promote urination, invigorate (tonify) the Spleen and calm the mind?
A. Zhu Ling(umbellatus)
B. Fu Ling(poria)
C. Ze Xie(Alisma tuber)
D. Yi Yi Ren(Coix seed)

2. Ze Xie (Rhizoma Alismatis Orientalis) has the following functions?
A. Promoting urination and expelling Wind-Damp to relieve pain.
B. Promoting urination and expelling Heat from the lower -Jiao
C. Expelling Wind-Dampness to relieve pain
D. Promoting urination and tonifying the Spleen.

3. All of the following herbs can clear Kidney deficient Heat, EXCEPT which of the following?
A. Ze Xie (Rhizoma Alismatis Orientalis)
B. Zhi Mu (Rhizoma Anemarrhenae Asphodeloidis)
C. Fu Ling (Sclerotium Poriae Cocos)
D. Huang Bai (Cortex Phellodendri)

4. Which of the following herbs is the best for edema with the Spleen Deficiency?
A. Mu Tong (Caulis Mutong)
B. Zhu Ling (Sclerotium Polypori Umbellati)
C. Yi Yi Ren (Semen Coicis Lachryma-jobi)
D. Ze Xie (Rhizoma Alismatis Orientalis)

5. Which of the following herbs can promote lactation?
A. Mu Tong (Caulis Mutong)
B. Zhu Ling (Sclerotium Polypori Umbellati)
C. Fu Ling (Sclerotium Poriae Cocos)
D. Yi Yi Ren (Semen Coicis Lachryma-jobi)

6. Which of the following herbs is the best to tonify Spleen and drain Dampness for diarrhea due to Spleen deficiency with Dampness?
A. Mu Tong (Caulis Mutong)
B. Ze Xie (Rhizoma Alismatis Orientalis)
C. Zhu Ling (Sclerotium Polypori Umbellati)
D. Fu Ling (Sclerotium Poriae Cocos)

7. Which of the following herbs is not marked as toxic but can cause renal failure if large dosage is used?
A. Guan Mu Tong (Caulis Aristolochiae Manshuriensis)
B. Yu Mi Xu (Stylus Zeae Mays)
C. Fu Ling (Sclerotium Poriae Cocos)
D.Yi Yi Ren (Semen Coicis Lachryma-jobi)

8. Which of the following herbs is commonly used for cancer and in the category of draining Dampness?
A. Yi Yi Ren (Coix seed)
B. Hua Shi (Talcum)
C. Ban Bian Lian (Herba Lobeliae Chinensis cum Radice)
D. Dong Gua Pi (Epicarpium Benincasae Hispidae)

Answer Keys: 1B. 2B. 3C. 4C. 5A. 6D. 7A. 8A

Section 2 Herbs that Benefit Urination and Treat urinary Tract Disorder

Indications:

Lin syndrome (including urinary tract infection, urinary calculus, prostatitis, chylous urine, urethral syndrome)

Herbs:

1. Che Qian Zi (Semen Plantaginis) 车前子
2. Tong Cao (Medulla Tetrapanacis) 通草
3. Di Fu Zi (Fructus Kochiae) 地肤子
4. Deng Xin Cao (Medulla Junci) 灯心草
5. Qu Mai (Herba Dianthi) 瞿麦
6. Bian Xu (Herba Polygoni Avicularis) 萹蓄
7. Shi Wei (Folium Pyrrosiae) 石苇
8. Bi Xie (Rhizoma Dioscoreae Hypoglaucae) 萆薢
9. Hai Jin Sha (Spora Lygodii) 海金沙
10. Hua Shi (Talcum) 滑石

Name	Property	CN	Actions & Indications	Remarks
Che Qian Zi (Semen Plantaginis) 车前子 Plantago seeds	Sweet Cold	BL KI LV LU	1. **Promotes urination:** for hot Lin syndrome, stone Lin syndrome and edema due to Damp-Heat; used with Mu Tong, Hua Shi. 2. **Stops diarrhea:** for diarrhea due to summer-Heat; used with Xiang Ru, Fu Ling. 3. **Brightens eyes:** for red and swollen eyes or blurred vision due to Liver and Kidney Deficiency or Liver channel Wind-Heat. A. Due to either Liver and Kidney Deficiency Used with Sheng Di Huang, Mai Men Dong and Gou Qi Zi. B. Due to Heat in the Liver channel.	5-15g **Wrapped** 1. Use with caution in cases of exhausted Yang Qi, or spermatorrhea due to Kidney Deficiency 2.Contraindicated for pregnant woman and a person without any

			Used with Ju Hua, Long Dan Cao. 4. **Clears Lung and expels Phlegm:** for cough due to Lung Heat; used with Jie Geng, Xing Ren.	Heat and Dampness symptoms.
Tong Cao (Medulla Tetrapanacis) 通草 Rice paper pith, tetrapanax	Sweet Bland Slightly Cold	LU ST	1. **Promotes urination:** for Lin syndrome and edema due to UB Damp-Heat; used with Hua Shi, Yi Yi Ren, Qu Mai. 2. **Promotes lactation:** for lactation Deficiency; used with Chuan Shan Jia, Dang Gui.	3-10g
Di Fu Zi (Fructus Kochiae) 地肤子 Broom cypress or kochia fruit	Sweet Bitter Cold	BL	1. **Promotes urination:** for hot type Lin syndrome due to UB Damp-Heat; used with Zhu Ling, Tong Cao, Qu Mai. 2. **Stops itching:** for Damp skin lesion such as vaginal itching, excessive vaginal discharge and eczema; used with Huang Bai, Ku Shen for eczema; used with She Chuang Zi for external vaginal itching.	10-15g Contraindicated in cases without Damp Heat.
Deng Xin Cao (Medulla Junci) 灯心草 Rush pith, Uncus	Sweet Bland Slightly Cold	HT LU SI	1. **Promotes urination:** for Hot Lin syndrome due to Damp-Heat; used with Mu Tong, Zhi Zi and Hua Shi 2. **Clears Heart:** for irritability, insomnia or infantile night crying due to Heart Fire disturbing Shen; used alone or with Chan Tui, Dan Zhu Ye.	**2-5g** Caution in case of Cold from Deficiency.
Qu Mai (Herba Dianthi) 瞿麦 Fringed pink (d. superbus) or Chinese pink (d.	Bitter Cold	BL HT SI	1. **Promotes urination:** for hot and stone Lin syndrome due to Damp-Heat; used with Mu Tong, Che Qian Zi, Hua Shi (such as Ba Zheng San). 2. **Moves Blood:** for dysmenorrhea, amenorrhea due to Blood Heat and stasis; used with Dan Shen, Chi	10-15g Contraindicated for pregnant women.

chinensis) dianthus			Shao, Hong Hua.	
Bian Xu (Herba Polygoni Avicularis) 萹蓄 Knotweed, polygonum	Bitter Slightly Cold	BL	**1. Promotes urination:** for hot Lin and Bloody Lin syndrome due to Lower Jiao Damp-Heat; used with Hua Shi, Mu Tong, Qu Mai (such as Ba Zheng San). **2. Kills parasites and stops itching:** for Damp skin lesion and roundworm abdominal pain; used with Bing Lang, Fei Zi.	**10-15g** Overdose can cause dermatitis or gastrointestinal disturbance and drain the essential Qi.
Shi Wei (Folium Pyrrosiae) 石苇 Pyrrosia leaves	Slightly Cold	LU BL	**1. Promotes urination:** for Hot Lin, stone Lin and Bloody Lin syndromes; used with Qu Mai, Hua Shi, Dong Kui Zi **2. Cools Blood and stops bleeding:** for bleeding such as vomiting with Blood, uterine bleeding, epistaxis due to Blood Heat; used with Pu Huang, Di Yu. **3. Clears Lung and expels Phlegm:** cough due ; used with Bing Lang.	5-10g Caution in the absence of Damp Heat.
Bi Xie (Rhizoma Dioscoreae Hypoglaucae) 萆薢 Fish-poison yam rhizome, tokoro	Bitter Neutral	BL ST LV	**1. Promotes urination:** for cloudy Lin syndrome due to lower Jiao Dampness or Damp-Heat. **2. Clears Dampness:** for Bi syndrome due to Wind-Cold-Dampness or Wind-Heat-Dampness.	10-15g It is the most important herb for Gao Lin syndrome.
Hai Jin Sha (Spora Lygodii) 海金沙 Japanese fern, lygodium	Sweet Bitter Cold	BL SI	**Promotes urination:** for every Lin syndromes but especially good for Stone Lin and Bloody Lin syndrome. A. Hot Lin, with Gan Cao. B. Bloody Lin, with Niu Xi, Hu Po, Xiao Ji. C. Stony Lin, with Ji Nei Jin, Hua	6-12g **Wrapped**

			Shi, Jin Qian Cao. D. Cloudy Lin, with Bei Xie, Hua Shi. E. Edema, with Ze Xie, Zhu Ling, Fang Ji, Mu Tong.	
Hua Shi (Talcum) 滑石 Talcum	Sweet Bland Cold	ST BL	**1. Promotes urination:** for Hot Lin and Stone Lin syndrome due to Damp-Heat; used with Mu Tong, Che Qian Zi (such as Ba Zheng San) **2. Clears Summer Heat:** for summer Damp-Heat manifested as fever, thirst, dark urine; used with Gan Cao (such as Lu Yi San). **3. Absorbs Dampness:** for Damp skin lesion, eczema, prickly Heat due to Damp-Heat. (Topically sue) Used with Huang Bai or use along.	10-15g **Wrapped** 1. Contraindi-cated in the case of Spleen Qi Deficiency or spermator-rhea 2. Contraindi-cated in the case of deficient fluids due to a warm febrile disease. 3. Use with caution during pregnancy.

Practice 12

1. Che Qian Zi (Semen Plantaginis) should be:
A. Wrapped for decoction
B. Decocted first
C. Decocted later
D. Steeped

2. Which of the following urine promoting and dampness draining herbs can not only treat Lin syndrome and edema but also for blurred vision due to Liver channel Wind-Heat and coughing due to Lung Heat?
A. Che Qian Zi (Semen Plantaginis)
B. Hua Shi (Talcum)
C. Tong Cao (Medulla Tetrapanacis)
D. Deng Xin Cao (Medulla Junci)

3. Which of the following herb is used for treating Damp Heat strangury (Lin syndrome) and clearing Summer Heat?
A Hu Zhang (Rhizoma Polygoni Cuspidati)
B. Yin Chen Hao (Herba Artemisiae Scopariae)
C. Hua Shi (Talcum)
D. Chui Pen Cao (Herba Sedi)

4. Both Chuan Mu Tong (Caulis Clematidis Armandii) and Tong Cao (Medulla Tetrapanacis) can:
A. Disinhibit urination, free the flow of strangury, dispel Wind and free the flow of the network vessels
B. Disinhibit urination, free the flow of strangury, and stop lactation
C. Disinhibit urination, clear Heat, and free the flow of breast milk
D. None of above

5. Which of the following urine promoting and dampness draining herbs can treat insomnia due to Heart Fire disturbing Shen and infantile night crying?
A. Tong Cao (Medulla Tetrapanacis)
B. Deng Xin Cao (Medulla Junci)
C. Qu Mai (Herba Dianthi)
D. Bian Xu (Herba Polygoni Avicularis)

6. Which of the following urine promoting and dampness draining herbs can promote

urination to free the flow of strangury (Lin Syndrome) and move Blood to treat dysmenorrhea, amenorrhea?
A. Tong Cao (Medulla Tetrapanacis)
B. Deng Xin Cao (Medulla Junci)
C. Qu Mai (Herba Dianthi)
D. Bian Xu (Herba Polygoni Avicularis)

7. Which of the following urine promoting and dampness draining herbs can promote urination to free the flow of strangury (Lin Syndrome) and Kill parasites to stop itching?
A. Deng Xin Cao (Medulla Junci)
B. Deng Xin Cao (Medulla Junci)
C. Qu Mai (Herba Dianthi)
D. Bian Xu (Herba Polygoni Avicularis)

8. Which of the following herbs is better for stone Lin syndrome and hot Lin syndrome and also stops cough due to Lung heat?
A. Deng Xin Cao (Medulla Junci)
B. Bian Xu (Herba Polygoni Avicularis)
C. Shi Wei (Folium Pyrrosiae)
D. Bi Xie (Rhizoma Dioscoreae Hypoglaucae)

9. Which of the following herbs is the "king herb" for treating Gao Lin syndrome (Cloudy Lin)?
A. Bian Xu (Herba Polygoni Avicularis)
B. Shi Wei (Folium Pyrrosiae)
C. Bi Xie (Rhizoma Dioscoreae Hypoglaucae)
D. Hai Jin Sha (Spora Lygodii)

10. Which of the following herbs is not only used for all kinds of Lin syndrome but also good for treating stone Lin and Bloody Lin syndrome?
A. Bian Xu (Herba Polygoni Avicularis)
B. Shi Wei (Folium Pyrrosiae)
C. Bi Xie (Rhizoma Dioscoreae Hypoglaucae)
D. Hai Jin Sha (Spora Lygodii)

11. Which of the following herbs should be wrapped for decoction?
A. Hai Jin Sha (Spora Lygodii)
B. Hua Shi (Talcum)

C. Che Qian Zi (Semen Plantaginis)
D. All of them

12. Which of the following herbs is the best one for Damp skin lesion such as vaginal itching, excessive vaginal discharge, and eczema?
A. Qu Mai (Herba Dianthi)
B. Bian Xu (Herba Polygoni Avicularis)
C. Hai Jin Sha (Spora Lygodii)
D. Di Fu Zi (Fructus Kochiae)

13. Which herb is contraindicated for pregnancy?
A. Tong Cao (Medulla Tetrapanacis)
B. Che Qian Zi(Semen Plantaginis)
C. Qu Mai (Herba Dianthi)
D. All of the above

Answer Keys: 1A. 2A. 3C. 4C. 5B. 6C. 7D. 8C. 9C. 10D. 11D. 12D. 13.D

Section 3 Herbs that Benefit Urination and Treat Jaundice

Indications:

1. Jaundice (For hepatitis, hepatocirrhosis, cholelithiasis etc.)
2. Damp carbuncle
3. Eczema

Herbs:

1. Yin Chen Hao (Herba Artemisiae Scopariae) 茵陈蒿
2. Jin Qian Cao (Herba Lysimachiae) 金钱草
3. Hu Zhang (Rhizoma Polygoni Cuspidati) 虎杖
4. Chui Pen Cao (Herba Sedi) 垂盆草

Name	Property	CN	Main Actions & Indications	Remarks
Yin Chen Hao (Herba Artemisiae Scopariae) 茵陈蒿 Yinchenhao shoots and leaves, capillaris	Bitter Acrid Cool	LR SP GB ST	**Clears Damp-Heat:** 1. Jaundice due to Liver and gallbladder Damp-Heat; can be used for both Yin and Yang jaundice; 2. Eczema, Damp type carbuncles. A) Jaundice due to Damp Heat; used with Zhi Zi, Da Huang (such as Yin Chen Hao Tang). B) Jaundice due to Damp Cold; used with Fu Zi, Gan Jiang (such as Yin Chen Si Ni Tang).	**10-30g**
Jin Qian Cao (Herba Lysimachiae) 金钱草 Lysimachia	Sweet Bland Neutral	BL GB KI LR	**1. Clears Damp-Heat:** for jaundice due to Damp-Heat; used with Yin Chen Hao, Zhi Zi. **2. Promotes urination:** for Lin syndrome, especially stone Lin; used with Hai Jin Sha, Ji Nei Jin. **3. Clears Heat and resolves Toxicity:** for carbuncle, burn, snake bite.	**30-60g**

Hu Zhang (Rhizoma Polygoni Cuspidati) 虎杖 Bushy knotweed root and rhizome	Bitter Cold	LR GB LU	1. **Clears Damp-Heat:** for jaundice, Lin syndrome, excessive vaginal discharge due to Damp-Heat. 2. **Moves Blood:** for amenorrhea, dysmenorrhea, injury, accumulations due to Blood stasis. 3. **Transforms Phlegm:** for Lung Heat coughing. 4. **Clears Heat and resolves Toxicity:** for carbuncle, burn, snake bite.	**10-30g**
Chui Pen Cao (Herba Sedi) 垂盆草 Sedum	Sweet, Bland, Slightly Sour, Cool	LR GB SI	1. **Clears Damp-Heat:** for jaundice due to Damp-Heat collecting in the Liver and Gallbladder. 2. **Clears Heat-toxicity:** for a variety of sores and abscesses, including those affecting the throat. Also used for snakebite and burns. Can be used alone for this purpose. Usually, the juice from the fresh herb is used.	15-30g

Practice 13

1. Which of the following herbs is the best for jaundice?
A. Yin Chen Hao (Herba Artemisiae Scopariae)
B. Jin Qian Cao (Herba Lysimachiae)
C. Hu Zhang (Rhizoma Polygoni Cuspidati)
D. Chui Pen Cao (Herba Sedi)

2. Which of the following herbs can treat stone Lin syndrome, jaundice and carbuncles?
A. Yin Chen Hao (Herba Artemisiae Scopariae)
B. Jin Qian Cao (Herba Lysimachiae)
C. Hu Zhang (Rhizoma Polygoni Cuspidati)
D. Chui Pen Cao (Herba Sedi)

3. Hu Zhang (Rhizoma Polygoni Cuspidati) has the following actions EXCEPT?
A. Clear Damp-Heat
B. Move Blood and transform Phlegm
C. Clear Heat and resolve toxicity
D. Brighten eyes

Answer Keys: 1A. 2B. 3D.

Chapter 5 Aromatic herbs that Transform Dampness

Common characteristics:

1. All of them are aromatic and most of them are warm.
2. Go to Spleen and Stomach channels.
3. Contraindicated in Yin Deficiency, use with caution for Qi Deficiency.
4. Do not decoct them too long.

Herbs:

1. Huo Xiang (Herba Pogostemonis) 藿香
2. Pei Lan (Herba Eupatorii Fortunei) 佩兰
3. Cang Zhu (Rhizome Atractylodis) 苍术
4. Hou Po (Cortex Magnoliae Officinalis) 厚朴
5. Sha Ren (Fructus Amomi) 砂仁
6. Bai Dou Kou (Fructus Amimo Kravanh) 白豆蔻
7. Cao Dou Kou (Semen Alpiniae Katsumadai) 草豆蔻
8. Cao Guo (Fructus Tsao-ko) 草果

Name	Property	CN	Actions & Indications	Remarks
Huo Xiang (Herba Pogostemonis) 藿香 Herba Pogostemonis or Agastache rugosa	Aromatic Slightly warm	LU ST SP	1. **Transforms Dampness, harmonizes the Middle Jiao:** for nausea, vomiting, abdominal distention, fullness, lack of appetite, diarrhea due to Dampness; used with Ban Xia, Cang Zhu. 2. **Releases the Exterior:** for Exterior syndrome with Dampness, Summer Heat, and Damp febrile disease; used with Zi Su Ye, Hou Po (as Huo Xiang Zheng Qi San). 3. **Stops vomiting; used** with Zhu Ru; Dang Shen, Bai Zhu; Sha	5-10g Do not decoct too long.

			Ren.	
Pei Lan (Herba Eupatorii Fortunei) 佩兰 Orchid	Aromatic neutral	ST SP	1. **Transforms Dampness:** for nausea, vomiting, abdominal distention & fullness, lack of appetite; used with Huo Xiang, Bai Dou Kou. 2. **Releases the Exterior:** for Exterior syndrome (Summer Heat) with Dampness; used with Huo Xiang, Qing Hao.	5-10g Do not decoct longer.
Cang Zhu (Rhizome Atractylodis) 苍朮 Atractylodes	Bitter Aromatic Warm	ST SP	1. **Dries Dampness, tonifies Spleen:** for nausea, vomiting, abdominal distention, fullness, lack of appetite, fatigue; used with Hou Po, Chen Pi (as Ping Wei San). 2. **Expels Wind-Dampness:** for Bi syndrome; used with Qiang Huo, Gui Zhi. 3. **Releases Exterior:** for external Wind-Damp-Cold. 4. **Improves vision:** for night blindness.	5-10g 1. Strong and good for Dampness in the Upper Jiao, Lower Jiao, interior, Exterior. Do not decoct longer.
Hou Po (Cortex Magnoliae Officinalis) 厚朴 Magnolia bark	Bitter Warm Aromatic	LI LU ST SP	1. **Transforms Dampness, moves Qi, removes stagnation:** for food stagnation, vomiting, abdominal distention, fullness, lack of appetite; used with Cang Zhu, Chen Pi (such as Ping Wei San). 2. **Improves bowel movement:** for constipation, ileus; used with Da Huang, Zhi Shi (as Xiao Cheng Qi Tang). 3. **Transforms Phlegm, directs Qi downward:** for cough, wheezing; used with Xing Ren,	3-10g 1; used carefully with pregnancy 2. Use with caution in cases of Qi Deficiency. 3. Do not decoct longer.

			Ban Xia, Xi Xin (as Gui Zhi Jia Hou Po Xing Zhi Tang).	
Sha Ren (Fructus Amomi) 砂仁 Cardamon	Aromatic Warm	ST SP	**1. Transforms Dampness:** for abdominal distention, fullness, nausea, vomiting, and diarrhea; used with Dan Shen, Bai Zhu. **2. Improves Qi and strengthens Stomach:** for lack of appetite, abdominal distention, fullness, pain. A. With food stagnation, Used with Mu Xiang, Zhi Ke, Bai Zhu (as Xiang Sha Zhi Shi Wan) B. With Spleen Deficiency, Used with Ren Shen, Bai Zhu, Fu Ling (as Xiang Sha Lu Jun Tang) **3. Calms fetus:** for morning sickness, restless fetus.	5-10g Do not decoct longer.
Bai Dou Kou (Fructus Amimo Kravanh) 白豆蔻 Round Cardamon Fruit, White Cardamon	Aromatic Warm	LU ST SP	**1. Aromatically transforms Dampness:** for abdominal distention, fullness, lack of appetite; used with Sha Ren, Hou Po, Chen Pi. **2. Warms the Middle Jiao and stops vomiting:** for nausea, vomiting; used with Huo Xiang, Ban Xia.	3-6g 1. Good for Upper and Middle Jiao. Do not decoct longer.
Cao Dou Kou (Semen Alpiniae Katsumadai) 草豆蔻 Katsumadai, Grass Cardamon	Aromatic warm	ST SP	**Dries Dampness and warms the middle:** for abdominal distention, fullness, vomiting, and diarrhea. A. Dampness obstructing the middle-Jiao, or with Qi stagnation, used with Sha Ren, Hou Po, Ban Xia. B. Vomiting, diarrhea due to	5-10g Do not decoct longer. Contraindicat-ed in cases of Yin Deficiency.

			Damp-Cold obstructing middle-jiao, used with Hou Po, Cang Zhu, Ban Xia with Rou Gui, Gan Jiang if severe Cold.	
Cao Guo (Fructus Tsao-ko) 草果 Tsaoko Fruit	Aromatic warm	ST SP	**1. Dries Dampness and disperses Cold:** for abdominal distention, fullness, vomiting, and diarrhea; used with Cao Dou Kou, Hou Po. **2. Checks malaria:** for malaria; used with Chang Shan, Hou Po.	3-6g Do not decoct longer; Stir-baked with ginger juice can reduce the possible side effect of vomiting.

Practice 14

1. Which of the following herbs has the function of transforming Dampness, warming the Middle Jiao, promoting the circulation of Qi, and calming the fetus?
A. Wei Ling Xian (Radix Clematidis)
B. Du Huo (Radix Angelicae Pubescentis)
C. Pei Lan (Herba Eupatorii Fortunei)
D. Sha Ren (Fructus Amomi)

2. Which of the following channels does Pei Lan (Herba Eupatorii Fortunei) enter?
A. Heart
B. Liver
C. Kidney
D. Spleen and Stomach

3. Which of the following herbs can dispel Wind-Dampness and be used for Bi syndrome?
A. Cang Zhu (Rhizoma Atractylodis)
B. Hou Po (Cortex Magnoliae Officinalis)
C. Pei Lan (Herba Eupatorii Fortunei)
D. Huo Xiang (Herba Agastaches seu Pogostemi)

4. If a patient has chills and fever without sweating, headache, abdominal pain, vomiting, a white greasy tongue coating, and a soggy pulse (Exterior syndrome due to Wind-Cold with Dampness in the Middle Jiao), which of the following herbs is the best to use?
A. Bai Hua She (Agkistrodon seu Bungarus)
B. Du Huo (Radix Angelicae Pubescentis)
C. Gou Ji (Rhizoma Cibotii Barometz)
D. Huo Xiang (Herba Agastaches seu Pogostemi)

5. Which of the following herbs is the best to treat Damp-Heat in the Spleen, marked by a sticky, sweet taste in the mouth, excessive saliva, and bad breath?
A. Gou Ji (Rhizoma Cibotii Barometz)
B. Cao Dou Kou (Semen Alpiniae Katsumadai)
C. Pei Lan (Herba Eupatorii Fortunei)
D. Cao Guo(Fructus Amomi Tsao-ko)

6. Herbs that aromatically transform Dampness should be decocted .
A. Early
B. Late
C. Separately

D. With wrapping

7. Which of the following herbs can promote Qi circulation and is commonly used to treat distention and fullness in the epigastrium and abdomen?
A. Cang Zhu (Rhizoma Atractylodis)
B. Hou Po (Cortex Magnoliae Officinalis)
C. Pei Lan (Herba Eupatorii Fortunei)
D. Huo Xiang (Herba Agastaches seu Pogostemi)

8. Herbs that aromatically transform Dampness are commonly used with herbs that
A. Regulate Qi
B. Dispel Wind to stop itching
C. Strengthen the tendons and bones
D. Clear deficient Heat

9. Which of the following herbs is the best for cough and wheezing with profuse, thin sputum due to Damp-Phlegm in the Lungs?
A. Cang Zhu (Rhizoma Atractylodis)
B. Hou Po (Cortex Magnoliae Officinalis)
C. Huo Xiang (Herba Agastaches seu Pogostemi)
D. Qin Jiao (Radix Gentianae Qinjiao)

10. Which of the following herbs can harmonize Middle-jiao and stop vomiting?
A. Fang Ji (Radix Stephaniae Tetrandrae)
B. Du Huo (Radix Angelicae Pubescentis)
C. Huo Xiang (Herba Agastaches seu Pogostemi)
D. Qin Jiao (Radix Gentianae Qinjiao)

11. Which of the following is NOT an indication of Cang Zhu (Rhizoma Atractylodis)?
A. Dampness obstructing Middle Jiao
B. Bi syndrome due to Wind-Cold-Dampness
C. Exterior syndrome due to Wind-Cold with Dampness
D. Blood stasis syndrome

Answer Keys: 1D. 2D. 3A. 4D. 5C. 6B. 7B. 8A. 9B. 10C. 11D

Chapter 6 Herbs that Dispel Wind-Dampness

Characteristics:

1. Most of them are acrid, bitter and dry.
2. May injure Yin and Blood.
3. Some are poisoning and should be used with caution.
4. Different properties and functions: warm or Cold or tonifying Liver and Kidney and strengthening bones.

Classification:

1. Herbs that dispel Wind-Cold-Dampness
2. Herbs that dispel Wind-Heat-Dampness
3. Herbs that dispel Wind-Dampness and strengthen bones and sinews

Common pharmacological functions:

1. Anti-inflammatory
2. Analgesic
3. Adjust immune function
4. Promote circulation

Cautions:

Caution with Yin and Blood Deficiency.

Section 1 Herbs Dispelling Wind-Cold-Dampness

1. Du Huo (Radix Angelicae Pubescentis) 独活
2. Mu Gua (Frutus Chaenomelis) 木瓜
3. Wei Ling Xian (Radix Clematidis) 威灵仙
4. Chuan Wu (Radix Aconiti) 川乌
5. Qi She (Agkistrodon) 蕲蛇
6. Wu Shao She (Zaocys Dhumnades) 乌梢蛇
7. Song Jie (Libnum Pini Nodi) 松节
8. Hai Feng Teng (Caulis Piperis Futokadsurae) 海风藤
9. Can Sha (Excrementum Bombycis Mori) 蚕砂

Name	Property	CN	Actions & Indications	Remarks
Du Huo (Radix Angelicae Pubescentis) 独活 Pubescent angelicae root	Bitter Acrid Warm	KI BL	1. **Expels Wind-Cold-Dampness and stops pain:** for Bi syndrome due to Wind-Cold-Dampness, especially for lower part of the body; used with Xi Xin, Qin Jiao, Qiang Huo. 2. **Releases the Exterior:** for the Exterior syndrome , Wind headache due to Wind Cold or Wind Cold Dampness; used with Ma Huang, Fang Feng.	3-10g **Use with caution for Qi and Blood Deficiency.**
Mu Gua (Frutus Chaenomelis) 木瓜 Chaenomeles fruit Chinese quince fruit Papaya	Sour Slightly warm	LR SP	1. **Expels Wind-Cold-Dampness and stops pain:** for Bi syndrome, spasm of tendons due to Wind-Cold-Dampness; used with Huo Xiang, Sha Ren, Bai Shao. 2. **Harmonizes Stomach:** for vomiting and diarrhea with abdominal pain due to Dampness blocking the Middle Jiao that leads to Qi ascending and descending disorder; used with Wu Zhu Yu, Xiao Hui Xiang, Sheng Jiang.	10-15g Excess taking can harm the teeth and bones.
Wei Ling Xian (Radix Clematidis) 威灵仙	Acrid Salty Warm	BL	1. **Expels Wind-Cold-Dampness and stops pain:** for Bi syndrome due to Wind-Cold-Dampness; used	5-15g 15- 30g for fish bone obstruction. Used with caution for weak patient.

Chinese Clematidis root			with Qiang Huo, Niu Xi. It can be used individually. **2. Expels Phlegm:** for Phlegm accumulation in the Middle Jiao. **3. Softens fish bone:** for fish bone obstruction in the throat.	
Chuan Wu (Radix Aconiti) 川乌 Prepared Aconite	Acrid Bitter Hot **Very Toxic**	BL	**1. Expels Wind-Cold-Dampness and stops pain:** for Bi syndrome, headache, body-ache, spasm of tendons due to Wind-Cold-Dampness. **2. Expels Cold and stops pain:** for Cold pain of abdomen, hernia and Cold extremities. It is a local herbal analgesic for doing simple operations or stopping pain due to injury.	3-9g **Decoct 30-60mins. Do not decoct longer. Contraindicated for pregnancy. Antagonistic with Xi Jiao (Cornu Rhinoceri) 犀角. Incompatible with Bei Mu, Gua lou, Ban Xia, Bai Lian, Bai Ji.**
Qi She 错误！未找到引用源。**/Bai Hua She** (Agkistrodon) 蕲蛇 Agkistrodon	Sweet Salty Warm **Toxic**	LV	**1. Expels Wind and unblocks channels:** for hard-treated Bi syndrome due to Wind-Cold-Dampness; stroke; used with Qiang Huo, Fang Feng, Qin Jiao. **2. Expels Wind and stop itching:** for leprosy, scabies, and another dermatosis. with Quan Xie, Wu Gong. **3. Stops convulsion:** for seizures, tetanus of pediatric patients. It is one of the best herbs to control convulsion; used with Quan Xie, Dang	5-15g as decoction and 1-1.5g as powder.

			Gui.	
Wu Shao She Zaocys Dhumnades 乌梢蛇 Black Striped Snake	Sweet Salty Neutral	LV SP	1. **Expels Wind and unblocks channels:** for Bi syndrome whether it is due to Wind-Damp-Heat or Wind-Damp-Cold, stroke, numbness of limbs; used with Qiang Huo, Qin Jiao. 2. **Stops itching:** for leprosy, scabies, and dermatosis; used with Chan Tui, Jing Jie, Chi Shao. 3. **Calms tremor and stops convulsion:** for seizures, tetanus of pediatric patients. It is one of best herbs to control convulsion; used with Bai Hua She.	5-10g as decoction and 2-3g as powder
Song Jie (Libnum Pini Nodi) 松节 Pine nodular branch	Bitter Warm	LR	1. **Expels Wind-Cold-Dampness and stops pain:** for Bi syndrome due to Wind-Cold-Dampness or pain caused by injury.	10-15g
Hai Feng Teng (Caulis Piperis Futokadsurae) 海风藤 Kadsura stem, Futokadsura stem	Bitter Acrid Slightly Warm	LR	1. **Expels Wind-Cold-Dampness:** for Bi syndrome due to Wind-Cold-Dampness; used with Gui Zhi, Wei Ling Xian. 2. **Unblocks channels and stop pain:** for pain due to injury.	5-15g
Can Sha (Excrementum Bombycis Mori) 蚕砂	Sweet Acrid Warm	LR SP ST	1. **Expels Wind-Cold-Dampness and stops pain:** for mild Bi syndrome due to Wind-Cold-Dampness,	5-15g **Wrapped**

Poop of baby silk worm			tendon or bone pain, rigidity of joints whether it is hot or Cold syndrome; used with Du Huo, Niu Xi. 2. **Transforms turbid Dampness and harmonizes Stomach:** for vomiting and diarrhea; used with Wu Zhu Yu, Hang Qin, Mu Gua. 3. **Relaxes spasm of gastrocnemius:** for spasm of gastrocnemius. 4. **Stops itching:** for measles, eczema; use topically or orally.	

Section 2 Herbs that Dispel Wind-Heat-Dampness

1. Qin Jiao (Radix Gentianae Qinjiao) 秦艽
2. Sang Zhi (Ramulus Mori Albae) 桑枝
3. Xi Xian Cao (Herba Siegesbeckiae) 豨莶草
4. Chou Wu Tong (Folium Clerodendri Trichotomi) 臭梧桐
5. Luo Shi Teng (Caulis Trachelospermi) 络石藤
6. Hai Tong Pi (Cortex Erythrinae) 海桐皮
7. Si Gua Luo (Luffae Fructus Retinervus) 丝瓜络

Name	Property	CN	Actions & Indications	Remarks
Qin Jiao (Radix Gentianae Qinjiao) 秦艽 Gentiana Macrophylla root	Bitter Acrid Slightly Cold	GB LR ST	1. **Dispels Wind-Dampness:** for Bi syndrome due to Wind-Dampness; used with Fang Feng, Du Huo, Qiang Huo, Zhi Mu, Ren Dong Teng. 2. **Clears deficient Heat:** for Deficiency Heat, steaming bone syndrome; used with Bie Jia, Qing Hao, Di Gu Pi. 3. **Reduces Dampness:** for	5-15g up to 30g Do not decoct longer or with high temperature. For any kinds of Bi syndrome. Best for Hot type.

			Damp-Heat jaundice; used with Huang Qin, Cang Zhu.	
Sang Zhi (Ramulus Mori Albae) 桑枝 Mulberry Twig	Bitter Sweet Slightly Cold	LR	1. **Dispels Wind-Dampness:** for both hot and Cold Bi syndrome due to Wind-Damp-Heat or Wind- Damp-Cold, rigidity of tendons; used with Guang Fang Ji, Wei Ling Xian. 2. **Promotes urination:** for edema.	**9-15g** **It mainly treats upper extremity Bi pain.**
Xi Xian Cao (Herba Siegesbeckiae) 豨莶草 Siegesbeckia Plant	Bitter Cold	KI LR	1. **Dispels Wind-Dampness:** for Bi syndrome. Good for Wind-Dampness in the bone and sinew. 2. **Resolves toxicity and clears Damp Heat:** for carbuncle and eczema. 3. **Reduces BP:** for hypertension.	10-15g Do not decoct longer if it is used for hypertension.
Chou Wu Tong (Folium Clerodendri Trichotomi) 臭梧桐 Glorybower leaf	Acrid Bitter Sweet Cool	LR	1. **Dispels Wind-Dampness:** for Bi syndrome due to Wind-Dampness-Heat, stroke, and numbness of limbs. 2. **Reduces BP:** for hypertension, especially hypertension with numbness of extremity.	5-15g Do not decoct too long if it is used for hypertension.
Luo Shi Teng (Caulis Trachelospermi) 络石藤 Star Jasmine Stem	Bitter Slightly Cold	HT LR	1. **Dispels Wind-Dampness:** for Bi syndrome due to Wind-Dampness-Heat, rigidity of tendons; used with Wu Jia Pi, Niu Xi, Ren Dong Teng. 2. **Cools Blood and reduces swelling:** for sore throat, swollen throat and carbuncle; used with Jie Geng, She Gan.	5-15g
Hai Tong Pi (Cortex Erythrinae)	Bitter Acrid Neutral	LR SP KI	1. **Dispels Wind-Dampness:** for both hot and Cold Bi syndrome due to Wind-Damp-Heat or	5-15g Higher dosage can cause

海桐皮 Erythrina bark			Wind- Damp-Cold. 2. **Kills parasites and stops itching:** for scabies, measles, and eczema; used both internally and externally.	arrhythmia and hypotension.
Si Gua Luo (Luffae Fructus Retinervus) 丝瓜络 Dried Vegetable Sponge	Sweet Neutral	LU LR ST	1. **Resolves Toxicity and reduces swelling:** for abscesses and other toxic sores. Often used for breast abscess, breast distention and lumps. 2. **Unblocks the channels and dispels Wind:** for Bi syndrome due to Wind-Damp-Heat or Wind-Damp-Cold, pain and soreness in the muscles and sinews, and stiffness in the joints, or chest and hypochondriac pain. 3. **Expels Phlegm:** for cough due to Heat in the Lungs with high fever, chest pain, and sputum that is difficult to expectorate; used in both adults and children. 4. **Promotes lactation**: for insufficient lactation.	6-10g up to 60g.

Section 3 Herbs that Dispel Wind-Dampness and Strengthen Bones and Sinews

1. Sang Ji Sheng (Taxilus chinensis (DC.) Danser) 桑寄生
2. Wu Jia Pi (Cotex Acanthopanacis) 五加皮
3. Qian Nian Jian (Rhizome Homalomenae) 千年健
4. Gou Ji (Rhizoma Cibotii Barometz) 狗脊

Name	Property	CN	Actions & Indications	Remarks

Sang Ji Sheng (Taxilus chinensis (DC.) Danser) 桑寄生 Mulberry Mistletoe Stem	Bitter Sweet Neutral	KI LR	1. **Dispels Wind-Dampness, strengthens sinews and bones:** for Bi syndrome with Kidney Deficiency and Cold, weak back and knee; used with Du Huo, Niu Xi, Ji Xue Teng. 2. **Calms fetus:** for excessive menstruation, for restless fetus; used with Xu Duan, Tu Si Zi, Huang Qi, Bai Zhu.	10-15g
Wu Jia Pi (Cotex Acanthopanacis) 五加皮 Acanthopanax root Bark	Acrid Bitter Warm	KI LR	1. **Dispels Wind-Dampness, strengthens sinews and bones:** for Bi syndrome with Kidney and Liver Deficiency and Cold, weakness of back and knee, child motor delays; used with Wei Ling Xian, Qiang Huo, Qin Jiao, Sang Ji Sheng, Niu Xi. 2. **Promotes urination:** for edema; used with Da Fu Pi, Fu Ling Pi.	5-15g
Qian Nian Jian (Rhizome Homalomenae) 千年健 Homalomena rhizome	Acrid Bitter Warm	KI LR	1. **Dispels Wind-Dampness, strengthens sinews and bones:** for Bi syndrome with Kidney and Liver Deficiency, weak back and knee, numbness of limbs.	5-15g
Gou Ji (Rhizoma Cibotii Barometz) 狗脊 Chain fern rhizome	Bitter Sweet Warm	KI LR	1. **Expels Wind-Dampness, strengthens sinews and bones:** for Bi syndrome & weakness of back and knee with Kidney and Liver Deficiency; used with Sang Ji Sheng, Gui Zhi. 2. **Controls urination:** for frequent urination and enuresis due to Kidney Deficiency, excessive vaginal discharge due	10-15g

			to Chong and Ren Deficiency Cold; used with Du Zhong, Niu Xi.	

Practice 15

1. Which herb can dispel Wind-Dampness and also release the Exterior?
A. Qin Jiao (Radix Gentianae Macrophyllae)
B. Sang Zhi (Ramulus Mori Albi)
C. Du Huo (Radix Angelicae Pubescentis)
D. Wei Ling Xian (Radix Clematidis Chinensis)

2. Which herb is especially used for pain of the feet or lumbar region and leg due to Wind-Cold-Dampness Bi?
A. Sang Ji Sheng (Taxilus chinensis (DC.) Danser)
B. Du Huo (Radix Angelicae Pubescentis)
C. Qiang Huo (Rhizoma et Radix Notopterygii)
D. Fang Feng (Radix Ledebouriellae)

3. Which herb can expel Wind-Damp, tonify LV and KD and strengthen sinews and bones?
A. Chen Pi (Pericarpium Citri Reticulatae)
B. Da Fu Pi (Pericarpium Arecae Catechu)
C. Sheng Jiang Pi (Ginger peel)
D. Wu Jia Pi (Cotex Acanthopanacis)

4. Which herb is for Bi syndrome with Heat, red and swollen joints?
A. Qin Jiao (Radix Gentianae Macrophyllae)
B. Du Huo (Radix Angelicae Pubescentis)
C. Wei Ling Xian (Radix Clematidis Chinensis)
D. Wu Jia Pi (Cotex Acanthopanacis)

5. What is the caution of using Mu Gua?
A. Food stagnation
B. Spasm and cramping of calves
C. Excess taking can harm the teeth and bones
D. Turbid Damp in the Middle

6. Which herb unblock the channels, extinguishes Wind and dispels Wind from the skin?
A. Bai Hua She (Agkistrodon)
B. Wu Jia Pi (Cotex Acanthopanacis)
C. Xu Duan (Radix Dipsaci Asperi)
D. Gou Ji (Fructus Lycii)

7. Du Huo (Radix Angelicae Pubescentis) gathers in or enters which channels:
A. Kidney, Heart
B. Kidney, Bladder
C. Kidney, Liver
D. Bladder, Gallbladder

8. Wei Ling Xian (Radix Clematidis Chinensis) should be combined with____ for Wind Damp impediment pain in the lower extremities:
A. Qiang Huo (Radix Et Rhizoma Notoptergyii)
B. Du Huo (Radix Angelicae Pubescentis)
C. Shu Di (Cooked Radix Rehmanniae)
D. Niu Xi (Radix Ahyranthis Bidentatae)

9. Which herb mainly treats upper extremity Bi pain?
A. Sang Ye (Folium Mori Albi)
B. Sang Bai Pi (Cortex Radicis Mori Albi)
C. Sang Zhi (Ramulus Mori Albi)
D. Sang Ji Sheng (Taxilus chinensis (DC.) Danser)

10. Which of the following medicinals treat both vomit and diarrhea and muscle spasms?
A. Huang Lian (Rhizoma Coptidis Chinensis)
B. Wu Zhu Yu (Fructus Evodiae Rutecarpae)
C. Mu Gua (Fructus Chaenomelis Lagenariae)
D. Ban Xia(Rhizoma Pinelliae Ternatae)

11. All of the following medicinals dispel Wind Dampness and are cool or Cold in nature EXCEPT:
A. Fang Ji (Radix Stephaniae Tetrandrae)
B. Qin Jiao (Radix Gentianae Macrophyllae)
C. Xi Xian Cao (Herba Siegesbeckiae)
D. Xi Xin (Herbal Asari Cum Radice)

Answer Keys: 1C. 2B. 3D. 4A. 5C. 6A. 7B. 8D. 9C. 10C. 11D

Chapter 7 Herbs that Move and Regulate Qi

Types Qi disorder:

1. Deficiency
2. Stagnation
3. Abnormally up or down

Qi stagnation related organs:

1. Liver
2. Spleen
3. Stomach
4. Lung

Common characteristics:

1. Most of them are acrid, aromatic, dry and warm and consume Qi and Yin.
2. Should be careful for Qi and Yin Deficiency.
3. Use with caution for pregnant women.
4. Contains volatile oil and should not be boiled longer.

Herbs:

1. Chen Pi (Pericarpium Citri Reticulatae) 陈皮
2. Qing Pi (Pericarpium Citri Reticulatae Viride) 青皮
3. Zhi Shi (Fructus Immaturus Citri Aurantii) 枳实
4. Zhi Ke / Qiao (Fructus Immaturus Citri) 枳壳
5. Mu Xiang (Radix Aucklandiae Lappae) 木香
6. Xiang Fu (Rhizoma Cyperi Rotundi) 香附
7. Chen Xiang (Lignum Aquilaiae) 沉香
8. Wu Yao (Radix Linderae Strychifoliae) 乌药
9. Tan Xiang (Lignum Santali Albi) 檀香
10. Chuan Lian Zi (Frutus Meliae Toosendan) 川楝子
11. Xie Bai (Bulbus Allii) 薤白
12. Da Fu Pi (Pericarpium Arecae Catechu) 大腹皮
13. Xiang Yuan (Fructus Citri) 香橼
14. Fo Shou (Fructus Citri Sarcodactylis) 佛手

15. Mei Gui Hua (Flos Rosae Rugosae) 玫瑰花
16. Li Zhi He (Semen Litchi Chinenesis) 荔枝核
17. Shi Di (Calyx Diospyri Kaki) 柿蒂

Name	Property	CN	Actions & Indications	Remarks
Chen Pi (Pericarpium Citri Reticulatae) 陈皮 Tangerine peel	Acrid Bitter Warm aromatic	LU SP ST	1. **Regulates Qi & tonifies Spleen:** for epigastric and abdominal distention, fullness, bloating, nausea, vomiting, loss of appetite. A. Accompanied with Dampness in the Middle Jiao, used with Zhang Zhu, Huo Po (as Ping Wei San). B. Accompanied with Cold and Stomach Qi rebellion, used with Sheng Jiang (as Ju Pi Tang). C. Stomach Qi rebellion and Heat, used with Zhu Ru, Sheng Jiang (as Ju Pi Zhu Ru Tang). D. Spleen and Stomach Deficiency, used with Dang Shen, Bai Zhu (as Yi Gang Sang). E. Diarrhea caused by Liver Qi attacking Spleen, used with Bai Shao, Fang Feng (as Tong Xie Yao Fang). 2. **Dries Dampness and transforms Phlegm:** for Phlegm-Damp cough; used with Ban Xia, Fu Ling, Gan Cao (Er Chen tang).	3-10g It can be divided into: **Ju Hong**—red tangerine peel **Ju He**—seeds, pip **Ju Luo**—pith, web **Ju Ye**--leaf **Hua Ju Hong**--Pomelo flavedo. . It can prevent the cloying nature of tonifying herbs from causing stagnation.
Qing Pi (Pericarpium Citri Reticulatae Viride) 青皮 Immature or green tangerine	Bitter acrid warm	G B LR ST	1. **Soothes Liver Qi:** for distention and pain in chest, breast and hypochondriac region, hernial pain. A. Bloating and pain in the hypochondrium, used with Chai Hu, Xiang Fu. B. Breast pain, used with Gua Lou, Xiang Fu.	3-10g

peel, blue citrus			C. Hernia pain, used with Wu Yao, Mu Xiang (as Tian Tai Wu Yao San). 2. **Removes food stagnation:** for abdominal distention, fullness, pain, used with Shan Zha, Shen Qu, Mai Ya. 3. **Dissipates clump:** for aggregation, accumulation, used with San Leng, E Zhu, Bie Jia, Xiang Fu.	
Zhi Shi (Fructus Immaturus Citri Aurantii) 枳实 Immature fruit of the bitter orange, chih-shih	Acrid bitter slightly Cold	LI SP ST	1. **Breaks up Qi & reduces accumulation:** for epigastric or abdominal pain and distention, constipation, diarrhea. A. Epigastric or abdominal pain and bloating due to food stagnation, used with Shan Zha, Mai Ya, Shen Qu. B. Epigastric or abdominal bloating due to Spleen and Stomach Deficiency, used with Bai Zhu (as Zhi Zhu Wan). C. Dysentery or diarrhea due to accumulation of Dampness, used with Da Huang, Huang Lian, Fu Ling, Ze Xie (as Zhi Shi Dao Zhi Wan). D. Constipation and abdominal pain, used with Da Huang, Mang Xiao, Hou Po (as Da Cheng Qi Tang). 2. **Transforms Phlegm and expels distention:** for fullness in the chest, used with Bai Xia, Xie Bai, Gui Zhi (as Zhi Shi Xie Bai Gui Zhi Tang)	3-9g Increase dose gradually; usually combined with Da Huang, Hou Po.

			3. **Raises organ prolapse:** for gastrectasis, gastroptosis, rectal prolapse, uterine prolapse, used with tonifying Qi herbs.	
Zhi Ke / Qiao (Fructus Immaturus Citri) 枳壳 Mature fruit of the bitter orange, chih-shih	Bitter Cold	SP ST	Same but mild in action than that of Zhi Shi.	3-10g
Mu Xiang (Radix Aucklandiae Lappae) 木香 Costus root, saussurea, aucklandia	Acrid bitter warm	G B LI SP ST	1. **Moves Qi and alleviates pain:** for abdominal pain and distention. A. With Huo Xiang, Sha Ren, Bai Dou Kou, Zhi Qiao (as Mu Xiang Shun Qi Wan). B. Accompanied with Deficiency of Spleen, used with Bai Zhu, Fu Ling, Gai Chao (as Xiang Sha Liu Jun Zi Wan). 2. **Regulates the Middle:** for diarrhea, tenesmus. A. due to Damp-Heat stagnated in the Stomach and Intestine, used with Huang Lian (as Xiang Lian Wan). B. due to food stagnation, used with Bing Lang, Zhi Shi, Da Huang. 3. **Moves Liver Qi and benefits gallbladder:** for epigastric pain and jaundice, used with Chai Hu. Yu Jin, Yin Chen Hao.	3-10g Usually combines with Da Huang, Bai Zhu. It can prevent the cloying nature of tonifying herbs from causing stagnation.
Xiang Fu (Rhizoma Cyperi	Acrid, Slightly Bitter,	SJ LR	1. **Moves Liver Qi:** for hypochondriac pain epigastric distention; used with Chai Hu, Bai	6-12g Main herb for Qi disorder and

Rotundi) 香附 Rut-grass rhizome, cyperus	Slightly Sweet, Neutral		Shao, Zhi Shi (as Cai Hu Shu Gan San). 2. **Regulates menstruation and alleviates pain:** for irregular menstruation and dysmenorrhea.	gynecological diseases
Chen Xiang (Lignum Aquilaiae) 沉香 Aloeswood, aquilaria	Acrid Bitter Warm aromatic	KI SP ST	1. **Moves Qi and stops pain:** for epigastric or abdominal pain and distention due to Qi stagnation with Cold or Spleen and Stomach Deficiency Cold; used with Wu Yao, Bing Lang (as Si Mo Tang). 2. **Guides Qi downward and harmonizes Middle Jiao:** for vomiting, hiccup due to Stomach Cold or Spleen and Stomach Deficiency Cold; used with Ding Xiang, Bai Dou Kou, Zi SuYe, Shi Di. 3. **Helps Kidney to grasp Qi:** for asthma, wheezing due to Kidney Deficiency not grasping Qi. A. Excess in the Upper Jiao and Deficiency in the Lower Jiao, with Su Zi, Ban Xia, Chen Pi (as Su Zi Jiang Qi Tang). B. Kidney can not receive Qi; used with Rou Gui, Bu Gu Zhi.	**1.5g-4.5** Contraindicated for Qi prolapse and Yin Deficiency
Wu Yao (Radix Linderae Strychifoliae) 乌药 Lindera root	Acrid Warm	BL KI LU SP	1. **Moves Qi and stops pain:** for epigastric or abdominal pain and distention, flank pain due to Qi stagnation with Cold. A. Fullness sensation in the chest, hypochondriac pain, used with Xie Bai, Gua Lou, Yu Jin. B. Epigastric and abdominal pain and distention, used with Mu Xiang, Wu Zhu Yu, Zhi Ke.	3-10g Caution in cases of Qi Deficiency or interior Heat

			C. Lower abdominal pain, hernial disorder, used with Xiao Hui Xiang, Mu Xiang, Qing Pi (as Tian Tai Wu Yao San). D. Menstrual pain, used with Xiang Fu, Dang Gui, Mu Xiang (Jia Wui Wu Yao Tang). 2. **Warms Kidney:** for frequent urination, enuresis due to Kidney Yang Deficiency; used with Yi Zhi Ren, Shan Yao.	
Tan Xiang (Lignum Santali Albi) 檀香 Sandalwood	Acrid warm aromatic	LU SP ST	1. **Moves Qi, warms the Middle and stops pain:** for vomiting and hiccup and abdominal pain due to Stomach Cold, chest pain due to Cold stagnated Qi in the chest.	**1-3g** in decoction. Added near the end.
Chuan Lian Zi (Frutus Meliae Toosendan) 川楝子 Sichuan pagoda tree fruit, sichuan chinaberry, melia	Bitter Cold **slightly toxic**	BL LR SI ST	1. **Moves Liver Qi, clears Heat and stops pain:** for hypochondriac pain and hernia pain caused by Liver Qi stagnation with Liver channel Heat; used with Yan Hu Suo (as in Jin Ling Zhi San). 2. **Kills parasites:** for roundworm, tapeworm and scalp tinea; used with Bing Lang.	3-10g. Can not use high dosage or long term.
Xie Bai (Bulbus Allii) 薤白 Bulb of Chinese chive, Macrostem onion, Bakeri	Acrid bitter warm	LI LU ST	1. **Unblocks Yang Qi, disperses Cold Phlegm:** for chest pain (Xiong Bi) due to Cold Phlegm obstructing chest Yang; used with Gua Lou Ban Xia (as Gua lou Xie bai Ban xia Tang). 2. **Moves Qi and reduces stagnation:** for dysentery. A. for Heat type; used with Huang Bai, Qin Pi.	5-10g. 30-60g when it is used fresh. Contraindicated in peptic ulcer.

			B. for Cold type, used with Huo Xiang, Shen Qu.	
Da Fu Pi (Pericarpium Arecae Catechu) 大腹皮 Betel husk, Areca peel	Acrid Slightly Warm	LI SI SP ST	1. **Moves Qi and removes stagnation:** for Stomach and Intestine Qi stagnation manifested as epigastric and abdominal distention and fullness, constipation or reluctant movement, regurgitation of food; used with Hou Po, Shan Zha, Mai Ya. 2. **Promotes urination and reduces edema:** for edema, urination retention; used with Fu Ling Pi, Chen Pi, Jiang Pi (as Wu Pi Yin).	5-10g Go downward
Xiang Yuan (Fructus Citri) 香橼 Citron Fruit	Acrid Slightly Bitter Sour Warm	LR LU SP ST	1. **Soothes Liver Qi:** for hypochondriac pain, chest distention due to Liver Qi stagnation. 2. **Regulates Qi and harmonizes the Middle:** for epigastric pain, poor appetite, belching and vomiting. 3. **Dries Dampness and transforms Phlegm:** for cough with chest pain due to Phlegm-Dampness.	3-10g Similar, weaker than Fo Shou, but good for transforming Phlegm.
Fo Shou (Fructus Citri Sarcodactylis) 佛手 Finger citron fruit	Acrid Bitter Slightly Warm	LR LU SP ST	1. **Soothes Liver Qi:** for hypochondriac pain, chest distention due to Liver Qi stagnation; used with Mu Xiang, Qing Pi, Zhi Ke. 2. **Regulates Qi and harmonizes the middle:** for epigastric pain, poor appetite, belching, vomiting due to Liver Qi overacting Stomach or Spleen and Stomach Qi stagnation; used with Chen Pi,	3-10g

			Huang Lian, Huo Xiang. 3. **Dries Dampness and transform Phlegm:** for cough with chest pain due to Phlegm-Dampness; used with Ban Xia, Fu Ling.	
Mei Gui Hua (Flos Rosae Rugosae) 玫瑰花 Young flower of Chinese rose	Sweet Slightly Bitter Warm	LR SP	1. **Moves Qi and relieves stagnation:** for Liver-Stomach disharmony manifested as abdominal distention or pain, nausea and vomiting, poor appetite. 2. **Moves Blood and stops pain:** for irregular menstruation, dysmenorrhea and injury.	3-6g
Li Zhi He (Semen Litchi Chinenesis) 荔枝核 Leechee nut	Sweet Astring-ent warm	LR ST	1. **Moves Qi, expels Cold and stops pain:** for 1. Hernial and testicular pain; 2. Abdominal and epigastric pain due to Liver Qi constraint; 3. Dysmenorrhea, post partum abdominal pain. A. Liver Qi stagnation syndrome, with Xiang Fu. B. Hernial or testicular pain due to Cold blocking the Liver channel, used with Ju Hua, Xiao Hui Xiang.	10-15g Powder is better
Shi Di (Calyx Diospyri Kaki) 柿蒂 Persimmon calyx, kaki	Bitter Astringe nt Neutral	LU ST	**Directs Qi downward and stops hiccup:** for belching or hiccup due to Stomach dysfunction.	6-10g

Practice 16

1. Which of the following not only dries Dampness and fortifies the Spleen but also dispels Wind Dampness?
A. Chen Pi (Pericarpium Citri Reticulatae)
B. Fu Ling (Sclerotium Poriae Cocos)
C. Bai Zhu (Rhizoma Atractylodis Macrocephalae)
D. Cang Zhu (Rhizoma Atractylodis)

2. Which of the following herbs has the functions of promoting the circulation of middle Qi, relieving pain and preventing the cloying nature of tonifying herbs from causing stagnation?
A. Mu Xiang (Radix Acuklandiae Lappae)
B. Shan Zha (Fructus Crataegi)
C. Qing Pi (Pericarpium Citri Reticulatae Viride)
D. Xiang Fu (Rhizoma Cyperi Rotundi)

3. A 30-year-old female complains of delayed menstruation, accompanied by distention and pain in the hypochondria and breasts, depression, a normal tongue, and a wiry pulse, which of the following herbs is the best to use?
A. Zhi Shi (Fructus Immaturus Citri Aurantii)
B. Da Fu Pi (Pericarpium Arecae Catechu)
C. Chen Pi (Pericarpium Citri Reticulatae)
D. Xiang Fu (Rhizoma Cyperi Rotundi)

4. Which of the following herbs is the best to prevent the cloying nature of tonics from causing stagnation?
A. Li Zhi He (Semen Litchi Chinensis)
B. Chen Pi (Pericarpium Citri Reticulatae)
C. Chuan Lian Zi (Fructus Meliae Toosendan)
D. Xiang Fu (Rhizoma Cyperi Rotundi)

5. A 69-year-old male complains of frequent urination with clear, copious urine, accompanied by Cold sensation in the lower back, a pale tongue with white, slippery coating, and a submerged, slow pulse, which of the following herbs is the best to use?
A. Zhi Shi (Fructus Immaturus Citri Aurantii)
B. Chuan Lian Zi (Fructus Meliae Toosendan)
C. Wu Yao (Radix Linderae Strychnifoliae)
D. Xiang Fu (Rhizoma Cyperi rotundi)

6. Which of the following herbs can soothe LV Qi, regulate menstruation and stop pain?
A. Xiang Fu
B. Chen Xiang
C. Chuan Lian Zi
D. Chen Pi

7. Which Qi regulator herb not only clears Damp-Heat but also kills parasites and treats skin diseases?
A. Mu Xiang
B. Chen Xiang
C. Tan Xiang
D. Chuan Lian Zi

8. Which herb is used for pain due to LV Qi stagnation?
A. Xiang Fu
B. Qing Pi
C. Chuan Lian Zi
D. All of the above

9. What is the function of Xiang Fu, Mu Xiang, and Wu Yao?
A. Descend rebellious Qi, and stop vomiting
B. Regulate Qi, and stop pain
C. Soothe LV Qi, and regulate Qi
D. Regulate Qi, activate Blood

Answer Keys: 1A. 2A. 3D. 4B. 5C. 6A. 7D. 8D. 9B

Chapter 8 Herbs that Stop Bleeding

Classification:

1. Herbs that cool Blood and stop bleeding
2. Herbs that move Blood and stop bleeding
3. Herbs that astringe and stop bleeding
4. Herbs that warm meridian and stop bleeding

Section 1 Herbs that Cool Blood and Stop Bleeding

Common characteristics:

1. Haemostatic
2. Cool or Cold
3. Antibiotic

Cautions:

1. Can not be taken longer
2. Dosage should not be too large

Herbs:

1. Da Ji (Herba Sue Radix Cirsii Japonici) 大蓟
2. Xiao Ji (Herba Cirsii) 小蓟
3. Di Yu (Radix Sanguisorbae) 地榆
4. Bai Mao Gen (Rhizoma Imperatae) 白茅根
5. Huai Hua (Flos Sophorae) 槐花
6. Ce Bai Ye (Cacumen Platycladi) 侧柏叶

Name	Property	CN	Actions & Indications	Remarks
Da Ji (Herba Sue Radix Cirsii Japonici) 大蓟 Japanese thistle, cirsium	Sweet Cool Bitter	LR SP	1. **Cools Blood and stops bleeding:** for bleeding caused by Blood Heat; used with Xiao Ji, Da Huang, Ce Bai Ye (as Shi Hui San). 2. **Reduces swelling and relieves toxicity:** for swelling,	10-15g. Fresh herb can be used up to 30-60g; used with Xiao Ji, Da Huang, Ce

			carbuncle and sore. 3. **Reduces BP and jaundice**	Bai Ye (as Shi Hui San)
Xiao Ji (Herba Cirsii) 小蓟 Small thistle	Sweet Cool Bitter	LR SP	1. **Cools Blood and stops bleeding:** for bleeding caused by Blood Heat. 2. **Reduces swelling and relieves toxicity:** for swelling, carbuncle and sore, use alone externally.	10-15g Similar but not as strong as Da Ji. It is good at hematuria.
Di Yu (Radix Sanguisorbae) 地榆 Burnet-Bloodwort root, Sanguisorba	Bitter Cool	LR LI	1. **Cools Blood and stops bleeding:** for bleeding caused by Blood Heat. A. Hemafecia, hemorrhoidal bleeding due to Damp-Heat in Large Intestine; used with Huai Hua Mi. B. Metrorrhagia and metrostaxis due to Blood Heat; used with Sheng Di Huang, Huang Qin. C. Dysentery with Bloody stool; used with Huang Lian, Mu Xiang. 2. **Clears Heat and generates flesh:** for sores, ulcers; used alone externally. 3. **Promotes healing of burns:** for burns.	10-15g Unsuitable for large areas of burns.
Bai Mao Gen (Rhizoma Imperatae) 白茅根 Rhizome of woolly grass, Imperata, White grass	Sweet cool	LU ST SI BL	1. **Cools Blood and stops bleeding:** for bleeding, used alone or with other herbs. 2. **Clears Heat and promotes urination:** for Lin syndrome, edema. with Che Qian Zi, Mu Tong. 3. **Clears Stomach and Lung Heat:** for nausea, wheezing; used with Zhu Ru, Lu Gen.	**15-30g.** It is better to use fresh. When it is fresh or alone, the dosage can be up to 30-60g.
Huai Hua	Bitter	LR	1. **Cools Blood and stops**	10-15g

(Flos Sophorae) 槐花 Pagoda tree flower (bud), Sphora flower	Cool	LI	**bleeding:** for bleeding caused by Blood Heat; used with Ce Bai Ye, Zhi Ke (Huai Hua San). 2. **Clears Liver and brightens eyes:** for red eyes and headache due to Liver Fire flaring up; used with Xia Ku Cao, Ju Hua.	This herb can lower blood pressure.
Ce Bai Ye (Cacumen Platycladi) 侧柏叶 Leafy twig of arborvitae, Biota leaves	Bitter Astringent Slightly Cold	SP LR LV	1. **Cools Blood and stops bleeding:** for bleeding caused by Blood Heat; used with Sheng Di Huang, He Ye, Ai Ye (Si Sheng Wan). 2. **Stops cough and expels Phlegm:** for cough due to Phlegm Heat. 3. **Promotes healing of burn** (use fresh form of herb): for burns.	10-15g Long-term use or a large dose may cause dizziness, nausea, vomiting.

Section 2 Herbs that Move Blood and Stop Bleeding

Common characters:

1. Hemostatic
2. Promote Blood circulation and remove Blood stasis
3. Some of them can decrease Blood lipid and cholesterol

Herbs:

1. San Qi (Radix Notoginseng) 三七
2. Qian Cao (Radix Rubiae) 茜草
3. Pu Huang (Pollen Typnae) 蒲黄
4. Jiang Xiang (Lignum Dalbergiae Odoriferae) 降香
5. Hua Rui Shi (Ophicalcitum) 花蕊石

Name	Property	CN	Actions & Indications	Remarks

San Qi (Radix Notoginseng) 三七 Rotoginseng root or Pseudoginseng root	Sweet Slightly Bitter Warm	LR ST LI	1. **Removes Blood stasis and stops bleeding:** for bleeding; use alone or with Xue Yu Tan 2. **Reduces swelling and alleviates pain:** for injury; used alone or with Ru Xiang, Mo Yao; used either orally or externally.	3-10g Contraindicat-ed in pregnancy.
Qian Cao (Radix Rubiae) 茜草 Madder root, Rubia root	bitter Cold	LR HT	1. **Cools Blood and stops bleeding:** for bleeding; used with Da Ji, Xiao Ji , Ce Bai Ye (Shi Hui San). 2. **Removes Blood stasis and regulates menstruation:** dysmenorrhea, injury, Bi syndrome; used alone or with San Qi.	10-15g Parched Qian Cao is better to stop bleeding. Raw Qian Cao is better to move Blood.
Pu Huang (Pollen Typnae) 蒲黄 Cattail pollen, Bulrush	Sweet Acrid neutral	LR HT SP	1. **Stops bleeding:** for bleeding; used alone or with Xian He Cao, Ce Bai Ye. 2. **Removes Blood stasis:** for chest, gastric, post partum pain and dysmenorrhea, used with Wu Ling Zhi (Shi Xiao San). 3. **Promotes urination:** for Bloody Lin syndrome.	3-10g Wrapped
Jiang Xiang (Lignum Dalbergiae Odoriferae) 降香 Dalbergia Heartwood	Acrid warm	LR ST SP	1. **Removes Blood stasis and stops bleeding:** for bleeding. 2. **Moves Qi and Blood, stops pain:** for chest pain, hypochondriac pain, gastric pain, injury.	3-6g
Hua Rui Shi (Ophicalcitum) 花蕊石 ophicalcitum	Sour Astringent Neutral	LR	1. **Astringes and stops bleeding:** for bleeding. 2. **Removes Blood stasis:** for injury	10-15g

Section 3 Herbs that Astringe and Stop Bleeding

Common characteristics:

1. Haemostatic
2. Astringent
3. Some of them are carbonized

Cautions:

1. Contraindicated in bleeding caused by Blood stagnation and excess pathogen
2. Can not be taken longer
3. Dosage should not be too large

Herbs:

1. Bai Ji (Rhizoma Bletillae) 白芨
2. Xian He Cao (Herba Agrimoniae Pilosae) 仙鹤草
3. Zi Zhu (Folium Callicarpae) 紫珠
4. Zong Lu Pi/Tan (Petiolus Trachycarpi) 棕榈炭
5. Xue Yu Tan (Crinis Carbonisatus) 血余炭
6. Ou Jie (Nodus Nelumbinis Rhizomatis) 藕节
7. Lian Fang (Receptaculum Nelumbinis) 莲房
8. Hua Sheng Yi (Pellis Seminis Arachidis Hypogaeac) 花生衣

Name	Property	CN	Actions & Indications	Remarks
Bai Ji (Rhizoma Bletillae) 白芨 Bletilla Rhizome	Bitter Sweet Cool	LU ST LR	1. **Stops bleeding:** for Lung and Stomach bleeding. Now it is used for TB and Stomach ulcer. A. Hemoptysis, used alone or with Pi Ba Ye, Ou Jie, E Jiao. B. Hematemesis, used with Wu Zei Gu. 2. **Reduces swelling and regenerates flesh:** for sores, carbuncles, chapped skin. A. Non-ulcerated sores,	3-10g Use as powder. **Incompatible with Wu Tou.**

			carbuncles, used with Jin Yin Hua, Bei Mu, Tian Hua Fen. B. Chronic non-healing ulcers, used alone for topical use C. Chapped skin, used alone or with Bai Zhi for topical use.	
Xian He Cao (Herba Agrimoniae Pilosae) 仙鹤草 Agrimony	Bitter Acrid Neutral	LU LR SP	1. **Stops bleeding:** for many kinds of bleeding based on combination with other herbs A. Heat syndrome, used with Huai Hua, Di Yu. B. Cold syndrome, used with Zao Xin Tu, Pao Jiang. 2. **Tonifies weakness:** for fatigue due to overstrain, used with Ma Chi Xian. 3. **Stops diarrhea and dysentery:** diarrhea and dysentery. 4. **Kills parasites:** for malaria, trichomoniasis, vaginitis, and tapeworm, used alone or with Ku Shen, She Chuang Zi.	10-15g Topical washing for trichomonas vaginitis.
Zi Zhu (Folium Callicarpae) 紫珠 Callicarpa leaf	Bitter Neutral	LU ST SI BL	1. **Cools Blood, Stops bleeding:** for wide variety of internal and external bleeding. 2. **Clears Heat and resolves toxicity:** for burn, sores.	10-15g
Zong Lu Tan/Pi (Petiolus Trachycarpi) 棕榈炭/皮 Trachycarpus stiple fiber	Bitter Astringent Neutral	LR LI LU SP	1. **Stops bleeding:** for variety of hemorrhagic diseases. 2. **Stops diarrhea and dysentery:** for diarrhea and dysentery.	10-15g Contraindicat-ed for pregnancy.
Xue Yu Tan (Crinis Carbonisatus)	Bitter Neutral	HT LR KI	1. **Stops bleeding, and removes Blood stasis:** for various type of bleeding.	5-10g

血余炭 Charred human hair			2. **Promotes urination:** for urination retention, Lin syndrome, especially Bloody Lin.	
Ou Jie (Nodus Nelumbinis Rhizomatis) 藕节 Node of the Lotus rhizome	Sweet Astringent neutral	LU LR ST	1. **Stops bleeding and removes Blood stasis:** for various type of bleeding.	10-30g Its action is weak. Usually used with other herbs.
Lian Fang (Receptaculum Nelumbinis) 莲房 Mature lotus receptacle, Lotus peduncle	Bitter Astringent Warm	LR SP KI	1. **Stops bleeding and breaks up Blood stasis:** for hemorrhagic diseases.	3-10g
Hua Sheng Yi Pellis Seminis Arachidis Hypogaeac 花生衣 Peanut peel	Sweet Bitter Astringent Neutral	SP LU	1. **Stops bleeding:** for inner organs bleeding, operation bleeding, haemophilia, thrombocytopenic purpura, and hemophilioid disease.	10-30g Its action is weak. Usually used with other herbs.

Section 4 Herbs that Warm Meridians and Stop Bleeding

Common characteristics:

1. Haemostatic
2. Warm

Cautions:

Contraindicated in bleeding caused by Heat.

Herbs

1. Ai Ye (Folium Artemisiae Argyi) 艾叶
2. Pao Jiang (Rhizoma Zingiberis Preparata) 炮姜
3. Fu Long Gan / Zao Xin Tu (Terra Flava Usta) 伏龙肝/灶心土

Name	Property	CN	Actions & Indications	Remarks
Ai Ye (Folium Artemisiae Argyi) 艾叶 Mugwort leaf, Artemesia	Bitter Acrid Warm	SP LR KI	**1. Warms the womb and stops bleeding:** for prolonged menstrual bleeding and uterine bleeding; used with E Jiao, Dang Gui, Bai Shao (as Jiao Ai Tang). **2. Warms womb and calms fetus:** for restless fetus; used with Xiang Fu, Rou Gui, Wu Zhu Yu (As Ai Fu Nuan Gong Wan). **3. Disperses Cold and alleviate pain:** for abdominal pain. **4. Expels Dampness and stops itching:** for diarrhea, leukorrhea, eczema, scabies. **5. Stops cough and wheezing:** for cough and wheezing.	3-15g
Pao Jiang	Bitter	SP	**1. Warms channel and stops**	3-6g

(Rhizoma Zingiberis Preparata) 炮姜 Quick-fried Ginger	Astringent Warm	LV	**bleeding:** for bleeding due to Spleen Yang Deficiency, in which Spleen does not control Blood. 2. **Warms the Middle, stops pain and stops diarrhea:** for abdominal pain, diarrhea due to the Middle Jiao Cold.	
Fu Long Gan / Zao Xin Tu (Terra Flava Usta) 伏龙肝/灶心土 Ignited yellow earth	Acrid warm	SP ST	1. **Warms the Middle and stops bleeding:** for bleeding due to Spleen Deficiency Cold, for dysfunctional uterine bleeding 2. **Warms Stomach and stops vomiting:** for Cold and Deficiency vomiting. 3. **Stops pain and diarrhea:** for chronic abdominal pain and diarrhea due to Spleen and Stomach Deficiency Cold.	15-30g Wrapped

Practice 17

1. The herbs in this category can stop bleeding through
A. Cooling Blood
B. Activating Blood
C. Astringing Blood
D. Warming channels
E. All of them

2. Which of the following statements is NOT correct?
A. Herbs that stop bleeding are only to treat symptoms. In clinical practice, they should be combined with different herbs according to different conditions (root causes).
B. Do not use cooling Blood alone if there is Blood stasis.
C. Massive haemorrhage usually accompanies escape of Qi, Yang and exhaustion of Yin. Thus, tonifying Qi, tonifying Yang and tonifying Yin herbs should be added at this condition.
D. Herbs that astringe blood to stop bleeding can be used for bleeding due to Blood stasis.

3. Which of the following herbs is the best for metrorrhagia and metrostaxis (uterine bleeding) due to Blood Heat?
A. Xiao Ji (Herba Cephalanoplos)
B. Da Ji (Herba seu Radix Cirsii Japonici)
C. Di Yu (Radix Sanguisorbae Officinalis)
D. Jiang Xiang (Lignum Dalbergiae Odoriferae)

4. Which herb is the best for treating traumatic injury with pain, bleeding and swelling with Blood stasis?
A. Da Ji (Herba Sue Radix Cirsii Japonici)
B. Xiao Ji (Herba Cirsii)
C. Di Yu (Radix Sanguisorbae Officinalis)
D. San Qi (Radix Notoginseng)

5. Which herb would you choose if a patient has bleeding and Blood stasis?
A. San Qi (Radix Notoginseng)
B. Di Yu (Radix Sanguisorbae Officinalis)
C. Huai Hua (Flos Sophorae)
D. Ce Bai Ye (Cacumen Platycladi)

6. Which herb would you choose if a patient has bleeding and Blood Heat?
A. San Qi (Radix Notoginseng)
B. Pu Huang (Pollen Typnae)
C. Jiang Xiang (Lignum Dalbergiae Odoriferae)
D. Da Ji (Herba Sue Radix Cirsii Japonici)

7. Which herb is especially good for bleeding from the LU (coughing up Blood) and ST (vomiting up Blood)?
A. Jiang Xiang (Lignum Dalbergiae Odoriferae)
B. Di Yu (Radix Sanguisorbae Officinalis)
C. Huai Hua (Flos Sophorae)
D. Bai Mao Gen (Rhizoma Imperatae)

8. What type of bleeding is most suitable for Di Yu (Radix Sanguisorbae Officinalis)?
A. Qi Deficiency
B. Blood stasis
C. Cold
D. Heat

9. Which herb can cool Blood, stop bleeding, and lower Blood pressure?
A. Di Yu (Radix Sanguisorbae Officinalis)
B. Huai Hua (Flos Sophorae)
C. San Qi (Radix Notoginseng)
D. Pu Huang (Pollen Typnae)

10. Which of the following herbal combinations can treat Blood in the stool and hemorrhoid bleeding due to Heat in the LI?
A. Ce Bai Ye (Cacumen Platycladi) + Xiao Ji (Herba Cirsii)
B. Di Yu (Radix Sanguisorbae Officinalis) + Huai Hua (Flos Sophorae)
C. Pu Huang (Pollen Typnae) + San Qi (Radix Notoginseng)
D. Huai Hua (Flos Sophorae) + Bai Mao Gen (Rhizoma Imperatae)

11. What is the function of Ce Bai Ye (Cacumen Platycladi)?
A. Cool Blood, stop bleeding, lower Blood pressure
B. Cool Blood, stop bleeding, expel Phlegm
C. Activate Blood, stop bleeding, promote urination
D. Warm channel, stop bleeding, calm fetus

12. What is the function of Bai Mao Gen (Rhizoma Imperatae)?
A. Cool Blood, stop bleeding, lower Blood pressure
B. Cool Blood, stop bleeding, expel Phlegm
C. Cool Blood, stop bleeding, promote urination
D. Warm channel, stop bleeding, calm fetus

13. Which of the following herbs should be wrapped for decoction?
A. San Qi (Radix Notoginseng)
B. Pu Huang (Pollen Typnae)
C. Qian Cao (Radix Rubiae)
D. Di Yu (Radix Sanguisorbae Officinalis)

14. Which herb can move Blood, stop bleeding, regulate menses?
A. San Qi (Radix Notoginseng)
B. Pu Huang (Pollen Typnae)
C. Qian Cao (Radix Rubiae)
D. Huai Hua (Flos Sophorae)

15. Which herb can move Blood, stop bleeding, promote urination?
A. Di Yu (Radix Sanguisorbae Officinalis)
B. Pu Huang (Pollen Typnae)
C. Qian Cao (Radix Rubiae)
D. Huai Hua (Flos Sophorae)

16. Which herb can move Blood, stop bleeding, move SP & ST Qi stagnation?
A. Di Yu (Radix Sanguisorbae Officinalis)
B. Jiang Xiang (Lignum Dalbergiae Odoriferae)
C. Qian Cao (Radix Rubiae)
D. Huai Hua (Flos Sophorae)

17. Which herb is especially good for bleeding from the LU (coughing up Blood) and ST (vomiting up Blood)?
A. Bai Ji (Rhizoma Bletillae)
B. Di Yu (Radix Sanguisorbae)
C. Bai Mao Gen (Rhizoma Imperatae)
D. Ai Ye (Folium Artemisiae Argyi)

18. What is the secondary function of Xian He Cao (Herba Agrimoniae Pilosae) besides being hemostatic?
A. Stop cough and expel Phlegm

B. Help healing the wounds
C. Promote urination
D. Stop dysentery and kill parasites

19. What is the function of Xian He Cao (Herba Agrimoniae Pilosae)?
A. Move Blood and stop bleeding
B. Astringe Blood and stop bleeding
C. Cool Blood and stop bleeding
D. Warm womb and stop bleeding

20. Which of the following herbs is best for the treatment of deficient Cold uterine bleeding?
A. Pu Huang (Pollen Typnae)
B. Huai Hua Mi (Flos Sophorae)
C. Di Yu (Radix Sanguisorbae)
D. Ai Ye (Folium Artemisiae Argyi)

21. Which of the following is NOT correct?
A. Bai Ji (Rhizoma Bletillae) can be used in cases of coughing of Blood with Exterior syndrome
B. Bai Ji (Rhizoma Bletillae) is incompatible with Wu Tou
C. Xian He Cao (Herba Agrimoniae Pilosae) may cause nausea and vomiting
D. Xian He Cao (Herba Agrimoniae Pilosae) can treat chronic diarrhea and dysentery with Blood.

22. Which of the following herbs can stop diarrhea and dysentery?
A Pu Huang (Pollen Typnae) + Huai Hua Mi (Flos Sophorae)
B. Di Yu (Radix Sanguisorbae) + Xian He Cao (Herba Agrimoniae Pilosae)
C. Xian He Cao (Herba Agrimoniae Pilosae) + Zong Lu Pi/Tan (Petiolus Trachycarpi)
D. Xian He Cao (Herba Agrimoniae Pilosae) + Zi Zhu (Folium Callicarpae)

23. Which herb can astringe, stop bleeding, remove Blood Stasis and promote urination, especially for Blood Lin syndrome?
A. Zi Zhu (Folium Callicarpae)
B. Xian He Cao (Herba Agrimoniae Pilosae)
C. Ou Jie (Nodus Nelumbinis Rhizomatis)
D. Xue Yu Tan (Crinis Carbonisatus)

24. Which herbs can not only stop bleeding but also break up Blood stasis?

A. Xian He Cao (Herba Agrimoniae Pilosae) + Zong Lu Pi/Tan (Petiolus Trachycarpi)
B. Ou Jie (Nodus Nelumbinis Rhizomatis) + Xue Yu Tan (Crinis Carbonisatus)
C. Ou Jie (Nodus Nelumbinis Rhizomatis) + Lian Fang (Receptaculum Nelumbinis)
D. Lian Fang (Receptaculum Nelumbinis) + Hua Sheng Yi (Pellis Seminis Arachidis Hypogaeac)

25. Which of the following herbs can warm channel to stop bleeding and warm the middle, stop pain and stop diarrhea?
A. Ai Ye (Folium Artemisiae Argyi)
B. Pao Jiang (Rhizoma Zingiberis Preparata)
C. Fu Long Gan / Zao Xin Tu (Terra Flava Usta)
D. Sheng Jiang (Fresh Ginger)

26. Which of the following herbs can calm the fetus through warming the uterine?
A. Huang Qin (Baical Skullcap root, Scutellaria)
B. Sha Ren (Cardamon Seed)
C. Sang Ji Sheng (Taxilus chinensis (DC.) Danser)
D. Ai Ye (Folium Artemisiae Argyi)

27. Which of the following herbs can warm the Middle to stop bleeding, warm Stomach to stop vomiting and stop diarrhea?
A. Hua Sheng Yi (Pellis Seminis Arachidis Hypogaeac)
B. Ai Ye (Folium Artemisiae Argyi)
C. Xian He Cao (Herba Agrimoniae Pilosae)
D. Fu Long Gan / Zao Xin Tu (Terra Flava Usta)

28. Which of the following herbs should be wrapped for decoction?
A. Fu Long Gan / Zao Xin Tu (Terra Flava Usta)
B. Pu Huang (Pollen Typnae)
C. Only A
D. Both A and B

Answer Keys: 1E. 2D. 3C. 4D. 5A. 6D. 7D. 8D. 9B. 10B. 11B. 12C. 13B. 14C. 15B. 16B. 17A. 18D. 19B. 20D. 21A. 22C. 23D. 24C. 25B. 26D. 27D. 28D

Chapter 9 Herbs that Move Blood and Remove Blood Stasis

Classification:

1. Herbs that move Blood and alleviate pain
2. Herbs that move Blood and regulate menstruation
3. Herbs that move Blood and treat injury
4. Herbs that move Blood and remove masses

Section 1 Herbs that Move Blood and Stop Pain

Common characteristics:

1. Most of them can move both Qi and Blood
2. Most of them contraindicated during pregnancy
3. They can be regarded as herbal pain killer

Herbs:

1. Chuan Xiong (Radix Ligustici Chuanxiong) 川芎
2. Yan Hu Suo (Rhizoma Corydalis Yanhusuo) 延胡索)
3. Jiang Huang (Rhizoma Curcumae Longae) 姜黄
4. Yu Jin (Tuber Curcumae) 郁金
5. Ru Xiang (Gummi Olibanum) 乳香
6. Mo Yao (Myrrha) 没药
7. Wu Ling Zhi (Faeces Trogopterori) 五灵脂

Name	Property	CN	Actions & Indications	Remarks
Chuan Xiong (Radix Ligustici Chuanxiong) 川芎 Szechuan lovage root,	Acrid Warm	LR GB PC	1. **Moves Qi and Blood, stops pain:** for Qi and Blood stagnation: 1. gynecological diseases; 2. hypochondriac pain; 3. chest pain; 4. stroke; 5. carbuncles with pus inside but not open; 6. injury. A. Menstruation, dysmenorrhea or	3-10g 1.It is Qi moving herb in Blood moving herbs 2. It is important

cnidium			irregular menstruation, with Tao Ren, Hong Hua, Dang Gui (as Tao Hong Si Wu Tang). B. Postpartum abdominal pain, used with Dang Gui, Tao Ren (as Shen Hua Tang). C. Hypochondriac pain, used with Wu Yao, Xiang Fu (as Ge Xia Zhu Yu Tang) D. Traumatic injuries, used with Chai Hu, Shan Jia (as Fu Yuan Huo Xue Tang). 2. **Expels Wind and stops pain:** for headache and Bi syndrome. A. Due to Wind Cold, used with Bai Zhi, Fang Feng, Xi Xin (as Chuang Xiong Cha Tiao San). B. Due to Wind Heat, used with Ju Hua, Shi Gao, Jiang Can. C. Due to Wind Dampness, used with Qiang Huo, Gao Ben, Fang Feng (as Qiang Huo Sheng Shi Tang). D. Due to Blood Deficiency, used with Dang Gui, Bai Shao. E. Due to Blood stasis, used with Chi Shao, Dan Shen, Bai Zhi. Bi syndrome (painful obstruction) A. Due to Wind-Damp in the Exterior, used with Qiang Huo, Du Huo (as Qiang Huo Sheng Shi Tang). B. Due to Wind-Cold with Kidney Deficiency, used with Sang Ji Sheng, Du Huo (as Du Huo Ji Sheng Tang).	herb for treating headache. There was a saying that "headache can not be treated without Chuan Xiong".
Yan Hu Suo (Yuan Hu) (Rhizoma Corydalis Yanhusuo)	Acrid Bitter Warm	HT LR ST LU	**Moves Qi and Blood, stops pain:** for all kinds of pain due to Qi and Blood stagnation.	3-10g It can "move Qi stagnation in the Blood, move Blood

延胡索/元胡 Corydalis rhizome				stagnation in the Qi, and stop any kind of pain everywhere in the body".
Jiang Huang (Rhizoma Curcumae Longae) 姜黄 Turmeric rhizome	Acrid Bitter Warm	SP ST LR	1. **Moves Qi and Blood, stops pain:** for chest and abdominal pain, injury with pain and swollen. A. Chest, hypochondriac pain, used with Chai Hu. B. Traumatic pain, with Hong Hua, Tao Ren. 2. **Moves Blood and unblocks menstruation**: for amenorrhea and dysmenorrhea; used with E Zhu, Chuan Xiong, Dang Gui. 3. **Expels Wind and unblocks channels:** it goes to the limbs for Bi syndrome; used with Qiang Huo, Dang Gui (Juan Bi Tang).	3-10g
Yu Jin (Tuber Curcumae) 郁金 Turmeric tuber, Curcuma	Acrid Bitter Cool	HT LU LR	1. **Moves Qi and Blood, stops pain:** for chest and abdominal pain; used with Dan Shen, Yan Hu Suo. 2. **Cools Blood and clears Heart:** for disorientation due to febrile diseases, epilepsy; used with Shi Chang Pu, Zhi Zi 3. **Benefits gallbladder and removes jaundice:** for jaundice, gallstone; used with Yin Chen Hao. 4. It is also used for vomiting Blood, epistaxis due to Liver Fire.	5-12g Antagonistic with **Ding Xiang.**
Ru Xiang (Gummi Olibanum) 乳香	Acrid bitter warm	HT LR SP	1. **Moves Blood and stops pain**: for chest pain, abdominal pain, masses, gastric pain due to Blood stasis, injury with pain and swollen, Bi	3-10g Important herb for trauma.

Frankincense, mastic			syndrome. A. Traumatic pain due to Blood stasis, used with Mo Yao, Xue Jie, Hong Hua. B. Chest, epigastric or abdominal pain due to Blood stasis, used with Dang Gui, Yan Hu Suo, Xiang Fu. 2. **Reduces swollen and regenerates flesh:** for carbuncles, sores, nodules, topically application for traumatic injury; used with Mo Yao, Xue Jie.	It is bitter and may cause vomiting.
Mo Yao (Myrrha) 没药 Myrrh	Acrid bitter neutral	HT LR SP	1. **Moves Blood and stops pain**: for chest pain, abdominal pain, masses, gastric pain due to Blood stasis, injury with pain and swelling, Bi syndrome. 2. **Reduces swelling and regenerates flesh:** for carbuncles, sores, nodules, topical application for traumatic injury; used with Ru Xiang, Xue Jie for topical use.	3-10g Can cause vomiting
Wu Ling Zhi (Faeces Trogopterori) 五灵脂 Flying squirrel feces, pteropus	Bitter sweet warm	LR SP	1. **Moves Blood and stops pain**: for gastric pain, abdominal pain, amenorrhea, dysmenorrhea and postpartum abdominal pain, fracture pain; used with Pu Huang (as Shi Xiao San). 2. **Removes Blood stasis and stops bleeding:** for uterine bleeding and retained lochia due to Blood stasis; used with Shen Di Huang, E Jiao. 3. Also used for childhood nutritional impairment; snake, scorpion and centipede bite.	3-15g. **Wrapped**. Antagonistic with **Ren Shen**

Practice 18

1. Which herb treats Bi syndrome and headache?
A. Ru Xiang (Gummi Olibanum)
B. Mo Yao (Myrrha)
C. Chuan xiong (Radix Ligustici Chuanxiong)
D. Dan Shen (Radix Salviae Miltiorrhizae)

2. What is the contraindication of using Chuan xiong (Radix Ligustici Chuanxiong)?
A. Deficient Yin with Heat signs
B. Headache from LV Yang rising
C. Qi Deficiency and excessive menstrual bleeding
D. All of the above

3. Yan Hu Suo (Rhizoma Corydalis Yanhusuo) is vinegar treated to ___
A. Enhance Qi regulating function
B. Enhance Blood activating function
C. Enhance analgestic function
D. Decrease toxicity

4. Which herb activates Blood, dispels stasis, cools the Blood, clears Heat and recedes or abates jaundice?
A. Yin Chen (Capillaris)
B. Zhi Zi (Fructus Gardeniae Jasminoidis)
C. Yu Jin (Tuber Curcumae)
D. Qin Jiao (Radix Gentianae)

5. Which herb if often combined with Shi Chang Pu (Rhizoma Acori Graminei) to treat Shen disturbance due to turbid Damp misting the HT orifices?
A. Chuan xiong (Radix Ligustici Chuanxiong)
B. Yan Hu Suo (Rhizoma Corydalis Yanhusuo)
C. Yu Jin (Tuber Curcumae)
D. Yi Mu Cao (Herba Leonuri Hterophylli)

6. Which of the following pairs of herbs activate Blood, reduce swelling and generate new tissue?
A. Tao (Semen Persicae) + Hong Hua (Flos Carthami Tinctorii)
B. Ru Xiang (Gummi Olibanum) + Mo Yao (Myrrha)
C. Sang Leng (Bur-reed rhizome or scirpus) + E Zhu (Zedoary Rhizome or Zedoaria)
D. Wang Bu Liu Xing (Semen Vaccariae Segetalis) + Chuan Shan Jia (Pangolin Scales, Anteater Scales)

7. Which of the following herbs can remove Blood stasis and stop bleeding?
A. Jiang Huang (Rhizoma Curcumae Longae)
B. Ru Xiang (Gummi Olibanum)
C. Mo Yao (Myrrha)
D. Wu Ling Zhi (Faeces Trogopterori)

Answer Keys: 1C. 2D. 3C. 4C. 5C. 6B. 7D

Section 2 Herbs that Move Blood and Regulate Menstruation

Common characteristics:

1. Move Blood and regulate menstruation.
2. Most of them are contraindicated for pregnant women.

Herbs:

1. Dan Shen (Radix Salviae Miltiorrhizae) 丹参
2. Tao Ren (Semen Persicae) 桃仁
3. Hong Hua (Flos Carthami Tinctorii) 红花
4. Yi Mu Cao (Herba Leonuri Hterophylli) 益母草
5. Niu Xi (Radix Achyranthis Bidentatae) 牛膝
6. Wang Bu Liu Xing (Semen Vaccariae Segetalis) 王不留行
7. Ji Xue Teng (Caulis Spatholobi)鸡血藤
8. Ze Lan (Herba Lycopi Lucidi) 泽兰
9. Yue Ji Hua (Flos Rosae Chinensis) 月季花
10. Chong Wei Zi (Leonuri Fructus) 茺蔚子
11. Lu Lu Tong (Liquidambaris Fructus) 路路通

Name	Property	CN	Actions & Indications	Remarks
Dan Shen (Radix Salviae Miltiorrhizae) 丹参 Salvia root	Bitter Slightly Cold	HT PC LR	1. **Moves Blood and regulates menstruation**: for dysmenorrhea, amenorrhea, irregular menstruation, postpartum abdominal pain; used with Dang Gui, Chuan Xiong, Yi Mu Cao. 2. **Moves Blood and stops pain:** for chest pain (coronary Heart disease), abdominal pain, masses, gastric pain, joint and limbs pain due to Blood stasis; used with Chuang Xiong, Chi Shao.	5-15g **Incompatible with Li Lu** (Radix Veratri).

			3. **Clears Heat and resolves carbuncles:** for carbuncles, boils, mastitis due to Heat. 4. **Clears Heart and soothes irritability:** for Heat entering Ying level, palpitation, and insomnia; used with Xi Jiao, Sheng Di Huang (as Qing Ying Tang).	
Tao Ren (Semen Persicae) 桃仁 Peach kernel, Persica	Bitter Sweet Neutral **Slightly Toxic**	HT LI LR LU	1. **Moves Blood and regulates menstruation**: for dysmenorrhea, amenorrhea, lochioschesis, injury pain, masses. A. Chest pain, used with Dang Gui, Hong Hua, Chuan Xiong (as in Xue Fu Zhu Yu Tang). B. Whole body ache or Bi pain, used with Niu Xi, Chuan Xiong (as Shen Tong Zhu Yu Tang). C. Amenorrhea, dysmenorrhea, used with Hong Hua, Chuan Xiong (as Tao Hong Si Wu Tang). D. Postpartum, abdominal pain, used with Dang Gui, Chuan Xiong (as Sheng Hua Tang). 2. **Expels pus:** for Lung abscess and Intestine abscess. A. Lung abscess: used with Yi Yi Ren, Dong Gua Ren for Lung abscess. B. Intestine abscess: used with Da Huang, Mu Dan Pi, Yi Yi Ren (as Da Huang Mu Dan Tang). 3. **Moistens Intestines:** for constipation due to dry	5-10g **High dosage can cause respiratory failure to death.** Usually combined with Hong hua.

			Intestines; used with Xing Ren, Chen Pi (as Wu Ren Wan). 4. Also stop cough and wheezing.	
Hong Hua (Flos Carthami Tinctorii) 红花 Safflower flower, carthamus	Acrid Warm	HT LR	1. **Moves Blood and regulates menstruation**: for dysmenorrhea, amenorrhea, postpartum abdominal pain; used with Tao Ren, Chuan Xiong. 2. **Moves Blood and stops pain**: for chest pain (coronary Heart disease), abdominal pain, masses, injury pain, nonsuppurative sores, carbncles. A. Chest or hypochondrium, used with Chi Shao, Tao Ren, Chuan Xiong (as Xue Fu Zhu Yu Tang). B. Hypochondrium, used with Chai Hu, Chi Shao. C. Traumatic injuries, used with Ru Xiang, Mo Yao. D. Sores, carbuncles, used with Pu Gong Ying, Lian Qiao. 3. **Moves Blood and resolves erythema:** for dark purplish erythema due to Blood Heat.	3-10g Contraindicated for ulcer patients Usually combined with Tao Ren。 High dosage can cause uterus spasm.
Yi Mu Cao (Herba Leonuri Hterophylli) 益母草 Chinese motherwort, Leonurus	Acrid Bitter Slightly Cold	HT LR BL	1. **Moves Blood and regulates menstruation**: for dysmenorrhea, amenorrhea, lochioschesis, and injury; used soft extract alone or with Chuan Xiong, Dang Gui, Chi Shao. 2. **Promotes urination and reduce swelling:** for edema with Blood stasis; used with Bai Mao Gen, Sang Bai Pi, Fu Ling.	10-30g

			3. **Clears Heat and resolves toxicity:** for boils, carbuncles, dermatitis.	
Niu Xi (Radix Achyranthis Bidentatae) 牛膝 Achyranthes root	Bitter Sour Neutral	LR KI	1. **Moves Blood and regulates menstruation**: for dysmenorrhea, amenorrhea, postpartum abdominal pain, injury; used with Chuan Xiong, Hong Hua, Chi Shao. 2. **Tonifies Liver and Kidney, strengthens sinews and bones:** for weakness of lower back and knee due to Liver and Kidney Deficiency, chronic Bi syndrome leading to Liver and Kidney Deficiency; used with Du Huo, Sang Ji Sheng (as Du Huo Ji Sheng Tang). 3. **Guides Fire/Blood down:** for vomiting Blood, epistaxis; headache due to Heat in the upper part of the body, dizziness and red eyes due to Qi and Fire rising or Blood Heat; headache, dizziness and red eyes due to Liver Yang rising; swollen gums, tongue and mouth sores due to Stomach Fire flaring up. 4. **Promotes urination:** for Lin syndromes and edema.	6-15g It can guide all herbs downward. Used with caution in cases with diarrhea due to Spleen Deficiency. **Chuan Niu Xi** 错误！未找到引用源。 is good at moving Blood. **Huai Niu Xi** 错误！未找到引用源。 is good at tonifying Liver and Kidney.
Wang Bu Liu Xing (Semen Vaccariae Segetalis) 王不留行 Vaccaria seeds	Bitter Neutral	LR ST	1. **Moves Blood and regulates menstruation**: for dysmenorrhea, amenorrhea due to Blood stasis. 2. **Promotes lactation and resolves abscess:** for insufficient lactation, mastitis. A. Due to Blood stasis, used	5-10g

			with Chuan Shan Jia, Tong Cao, Lu Lu Tong. B. Due to Qi Deficiency, used with Huang Qi, Dang Gui. 3. **Promotes urination:** for Lin syndromes including hot Lin, Bloody Lin, stone Lin. 4. **Used as ear seeds:** for auricular points.	
Ji Xue Teng (Caulis Spatholobi) 鸡血藤 Spatholobus or millettia root and vine	Bitter Sweet Warm	LR KD	1. **Moves Blood and tonifies Blood:** for irregular menstruation, dysmenorrhea, and amenorrhea due to Blood stasis or Blood Deficiency; used with Shu Di Huang, Chuan Xiong, Dang Gui. 2. **Relaxes sinews and unblocks channels:** for Bi syndrome, numbness of extremities, lower back and knee pain, joint soreness, stroke paralysis; used with Du Huo, Sang Ji Sheng.	10-15g Good at Blood stasis with Blood Deficiency.
Ze Lan (Herba Lycopi Lucidi) 泽兰 Bugleweed	Bitter Acrid Slightly Warm Aromatic	LR SP	1. **Moves Blood** and **regulates menstruation**: for dysmenorrhea, amenorrhea, and postpartum abdominal pain; used with Dang Gui, Yi Mu Cao, Shan Shen. 2. **Moves Blood and clears Heat:** for injury, chest and hypochondriac pain, boils and carbuncles; used with Chi Shao, Chuan Xiong, Ru Xiang. 3. **Promotes urination:** for post partum edema, post partum urinary retention.	10-15g Use with caution during pregnancy and in cases without Blood stasis.

Yue Ji Hua (Flos Rosae Chinensis) 月季花 Partially Opened Flower of Chinese Tea Rose	Sweet Warm	LR	1. **Moves Blood, regulates menstruation and moves Liver Qi**: for irregular menstruation, dysmenorrhea, amenorrhea, hypochondriac and abdominal pain. 2. **Reduces swelling:** for carbuncles, boils, scrofula, and injury.	3-6g
Lu Lu Tong (Liquidambaris Fructus) 路路通 Sweetgum Fruit	Bitter Neutral	LR ST	1. **Expels Wind and unblocks channels:** for Bi syndromes, injury. 2. **Promotes urination:** for edema. 3. **Promotes lactation:** for insufficient lactation, mastitis.	5-10g

Practice 19

1. Which herb can be used for Blood Heat stagnation and/or Blood Deficiency?
A. Yan Hu Suo (Rhizoma Corydalis Yanhusuo)
B. Dan Shen (Radix Salviae Miltiorrhizae)
C. Dang Shen (Radix Codonopsis Pilosulae)
D. Dang Gui (Radix Angelicae Sinensis)

2. Which Blood activator can promote urination?
A. Yi Mu Cao (Herba Leonuri Hterophylli)
B. Ze Lan (Herba Lycopi Lucidi)
C. All of the above
D. None of the above

3. Which of the following herb is best for Blood stasis abdominal pain and constipation?
A. Xin Ren (Semen Pruni Armeniacae)
B. Tao Ren (Semen Persicae)
C. Bai Zi Ren (Semen Platycladi)
D. Hu Tao Ren (Semen Juglandis)

4. What is the indication of Niu Xi (Radix Achyranthis Bidentatae)?
A. Weak knee, lumbago
B. Dysuria, painful urination
C. Hemoptysis, mouth ulceration
D. All of the above

5. Which of the following herbs can remove Blood stasis and stop bleeding?
A.Jiang Huang (Rhizoma Curcumae Longae)
B. Ru Xiang (Gummi Olibanum)
C. Mo Yao (Myrrha)
D. Wu Ling Zhi (Faeces Trogopterori)

6. Which of Blood-moving herbs can clear Heat and resolve carbuncles, clear Heart and soothe irritability?
A. Dan Shen (Radix Salviae Miltiorrhizae)
B. Hong Hua (Flos Carthami Tinctorii)
C. Tao Ren (Semen Persicae)

D. Yi Mu Cao (Herba Leonuri Hterophylli)

7. Which of Blood-moving herbs can invigorate channels and strengthen the sinews?
A. Yi Mu Cao (Herba Leonuri Hterophylli)
B. Ze Lan (Herba Lycopi Lucidi)
C. Niu Xi (Radix Achyranthis Bidentatae)
D. Ji Xue Teng (Caulis Spatholobi)

Answer Keys: 1B. 2C. 3B. 4D. 5D. 6A. 7D

Section 3 Herbs that Move Blood and Treat Injury

1. Su Mu (Lignum Sappan) 苏木
2. Zi Ran Tong (Pyritum) 自然铜
3. Gu Sui Bu (Rhizoma Drynariae) 骨碎补
4. Liu Ji Nu (Herba Artemisiae Anomalae) 刘寄奴
5. Ma Qian Zi (Semen Strychni) 马钱子
6. Er Cha (Pasta Acaciae seu Uncariae) 儿茶

Name	Property	CN	Actions & Indications	Remarks
Su Mu (Lignum Sappan) 苏木 Sappan wood	Sweet Salty Acrid neutral	HT LR SP	1. **Moves Blood, promotes healing of injury:** for traumatic injury, bone fracture and carbuncles. 2. **Moves Blood and stops pain:** for chest and abdominal pain due to Blood stasis. 3. **Removes Blood stasis and regulates menstruation:** for amenorrhea, dysmenorrhea, postpartum bleeding.	3-10g Contraindicated during pregnancy.
Zi Ran Tong (Pyritum) 自然铜 Pyrite	Acrid Bitter neutral	LR KI	1. **Reconnects sinews and bones, promotes healing of injury:** for traumatic injury and bone fracture.	10-15g
Gu Sui Bu (Rhizoma Drynariae) 骨碎补 Kolswaebo	Bitter Warm	KI LR	1. **Moves Blood and reconnects sinews and bones:** for traumatic injury, bone fracture with swelling and pain. 2. **Tonifies Kidney Yang:** for weakness of knee and lower back, tinnitus, deafness, toothache due to Kidney Yang Deficiency.	10-15g

Liu Ji Nu (Herba Artemisiae Anomalae) 刘寄奴 Artemesia	Bitter warm	HT SP	1. **Moves Blood, stops pain and stops bleeding:** for traumatic injury, bone fracture. 2. **Regulates menstruation:** for amenorrhea, postpartum abdominal pain. 3. **Improves digestion:** for food stagnation.	**10-30g**
Ma Qian Zi (Semen Strychni) 马钱子 Nux-vomica seeds	Bitter Cold **Extremely Toxic**	LR SP	1. **Unblocks channles and stops pain (Externally use):** for Bi syndrome, traumatic injury; used with Xiong Huang, Ru Xiang, Chuan Shan Jia. 2. **Disperses clumps, reduces swelling and stops pain (External use):** for carbuncle; used with Ru Xiang, Mo Yao, Zi Ran Tong, Gu Sui Bu 3. **For cancer.**	External use with proper dosage. Internal use 0.3-0.6g as powder.
Er Cha (Pasta Acaciae seu Uncariae) 儿茶 Catechu	Bitter Astringent cool	LU	1. **Moves Blood, stops bleeding, dries Dampness and absorbs seepage (External use):** for injury, carbuncle, and mouth sore. 2. **Clears Phlegm-Heat (Internal taken):** for coughing due to Phlegm-Heat.	External use with proper dosage. Internal use 1-3g Wrapped

Section 4 Herbs that Move Blood and Remove Mass

1. Tu Bie Chong (Eupolyphaga Seu Steleophaga) 土鳖虫
2. San Leng (Rhizoma Sparganii) 三棱
3. E Zhu (Rhizoma Curcumae) 莪术
4. Shui Zhi (Hirudo) 水蛭
5. Mang Chong (Tabanus) 虻虫
6. Chuan San Jia (Squama Manis) 穿山甲
7. Ban Mao (Mylabris) 斑蝥
8. Ling Xiao Hua (Flos Campsis) 凌霄花
9. Gan Qi (Resina Taxicodendri) 干漆

Name	Property	CN	Actions & Indications	Remarks
Tu Bie Chong (Eupolyphaga Seu Steleophaga) 土鳖虫 Wingless cockroach, eupolyphaga	Salty Cold **slightly toxic**	LR HT SP	1. **Reconnects sinews and bones:** for injury, laceration, contusion and fracture; used with Gu Cui Bu, Ru Xiang. 2. **Removes Blood stasis and regulates menstruation:** for masses and amenorrhea A. Abdominal masses, used with Chai Hu, Tao Ren, Bie Jia. B. Amenorrhea, used with Da Huang, Tao Ren (as Xia Yu Xue Tang).	3-10g
San Leng (Rhizoma Sparganii) 三棱 Bur-reed rhizome, scirpus	Bitter Acrid Neutral	LR SP	1. **Breaks up Blood and removes Blood stasis:** for abdominal pain, chest pain, dysmenorrhea, amenorrhea, abdominal mass. A. Amenorrhea, dysmenorrhea, post partum abdominal pain, used with E Zhu, Niu Xi, Chuan Xiong. B. Abdominal mass, used with Dan Shen, Yu Jin, Mu Li.	3-10g **Antagonistic with Ya Xiao**

			C. Pain and swelling due to trauma, used with E Zhu, Ru Xiang. 2. **Dissolves food accumulation and stops pain:** for food stagnation; used with E Zhu, Qing Pi, Chen Pi.	
E Zhu (Rhizoma Curcumae) 莪术 Zedoary rhizome, zedoaria	Acrid Bitter warm	LR SP	1. **Breaks up Blood and drives out Blood stasis:** for abdominal pain, chest pain, dysmenorrhea, amenorrhea, abdominal mass A. Dysmenorrhea, amenorrhea, used with San Leng, Dang Gui, Chuan Xiong. B. Abdominal pain and masses, epigastric masses, used with San Leng, Mu Xiang. C. Pain, swelling due to trauma, used with Chuan Xiong, Ze Lan, San Leng. 2. **Dissolves food accumulation and stops pain:** for food stagnation; used with San Leng, Mai Ya.	3-10g
Shui Zhi (Hirudo) 水蛭 Leech	Salty Bitter Neutral **Slightly toxic**	LR BL	1. **Breaks up Blood and drives out Blood stasis:** for dysmenorrhea, amenorrhea, abdominal mass, injury and fracture. A. Amenorrhea, immobile abdominal masses, used with Tao Ren, Hong Hua, San Leng. B. Traumatic injury: a. Pain, bone broken, used with Mo Yao, Su Mu. b. Internal Blood stasis, used with Da Huang, Qian Niu Zi.	**1.5-3g** as decoction and 0.3-0.5g as powder.
Mang Chong	Bitter	LR	1. **Breaks up Blood and unblocks**	**1.5-3g** as

(Tabanus) 虻虫 Gadfly Female	slightly Cold **slightly toxic**	ST	**channels:** for dysmenorrhea, amenorrhea, abdominal mass 2. **Moves Blood and stops pain:** injury and fracture.	decoction and 0.3-0.6g as powder.
Chuan Shan Jia (Squama Manis) 穿山甲 Pangolin scales, anteater scales	Salty cool	LR ST	1. **Breaks up Blood and drives out Blood stasis:** for dysmenorrhea, amenorrhea, abdominal mass and Bi syndrome. 2. **Promotes lactation:** for lactation Deficiency of nursing mother. 3. **Reduces swelling and promotes discharge of pus:** for carbuncle, nodules.	3-10g
Ban Mao (Mylabris) 斑蝥 Cantharides, mylabris	Acrid Cold **Extremely Toxic**	LI LR SI	1. **Resolves toxicity (External use):** for carbuncle, scrofula, mad dog bite. 2. **Moves Blood and removes mass (Internal use):** for amenorrhea, masses, cancer.	Internal use **0.03-0.06g.** External use with proper dosage.
Ling Xiao Hua (Flos Campsis) 凌霄花 Chinese trumpetcreeper	Pungent Acrid Cold	LV PC	**1. Moves Blood and removes stasis** **2. Cools Blood and extinguishes Wind**	
Gan Qi (Resina Taxicodendri) 干漆 Dried Lacquer	Acrid Bitter Warm **Slightly toxic**	LR ST	**1. Breaks up Blood and drives out Blood stasis** **2. Kills parasites**	

Practice 20

1. Which breaking-up herb can tonify KD and SP Yang, also can tonify LU and KD Deficiency?
A. Zi Ran Tong (Pyrite)
B. Su Mu (Sappan wood)
C. Gu Sui Bu (kolswaebo)
D. Ma Qian Zi (nux-vomica seeds)

2. Which breaking-up herb is extremely TOXIC and uses for Bi syndrome, carbuncle and cancer?
A. Zhe Chong (wingless cockroach, eupolyphaga)
B. Su Mu (Sappan wood)
C. Gu Sui Bu (kolswaebo)
D. Ma Qian Zi (nux-vomica seeds)

3. Which of the following pairs of herbs break Blood stasis for abdominal masses?
A. Tao Ren + Hong Hua
B. Ru Xiang + Mo Yao
C. Sang Leng + E Zhu
D. Wang Bu Liu Xing + Chuan Shan Jia

4. Which herbal combination can treat insufficient lactation due to Blood stasis?
A. Tao Ren + Hong Hua
B. Ru Xiang + Mo Yao
C. Sang Leng + E Zhu
D. Wang Bu Liu Xing + Chuan Shan Jia

5. Which of the following herbs is slightly toxic?
A. Shui Zhi (Hirudo seu Whitmania)
B. Ji Xue Teng (Tradix et Caulis Jixuteng)
C. Bai Mao Gen (Rhizome Imperatae Cylindricae)
D. Yi Mu Cao (Herba Leonuri Heterophylli)

6. Which of the following herbs has the functions of breaking up and driving out Blood stasis, renewing sinews and joining bones?
A. Zhe Chong (Eeupolyphaga seu Opisthoplatia)
B. Mai Ya (Fructus Hordei Vulgaris Germinantus)

C. Gu Ya (Fructus Oryzae Sativae Germinantus)
D. Lai Fu Zi (Semen Raphani Sativi)

7. Which of the following herbs not only can reduce food stagnation, but also break up Blood stasis, promote the movement of Qi and alleviate pain?
A. Shen Qu (Massa Fermentata)
B. Mai Ya (Fructus Hordei Vulgaris Germinantus)
C. San Leng (Rhizoma Sparganii Stoloniferi)
D. Gu Ya (Fructus Oryzae Sativae Germinantus)

8. Which of the following herbs can remove Blood stasis, reduce swelling, promote discharge of pus, and is the best for sores in both early and middle stage?
A. Mu Xiang (Radix Aucklandiae Lappae)
B. Chuan Shan Jia (Squama Manitis Pentadactylae)
C. Qing Pi (Pericarpium Citri Reticulatae Viride)
D. Xiang Fu (Rhizoma Cyperi rotundi)

9. What is the difference between San Leng (Rhizoma Sparganii Stoloniferi) and E Zhu (Rhizoma Curcumae Ezhu)?
A. E Zhu can reduce food stagnation, San Leng cannot
B. E Zhu can invigorate the movement of Qi, San Leng cannot
C. San Leng is stronger in breaking up Blood stasis
D. San Leng can alleviate pain, E Zhu cannot

10. Which of the following herbs are toxic?
A. Zhe chong (wingless cockroach, eupolyphaga), Chuan Shan Jia (pangolin scales, anteater scales)
B. Ma Qian Zi (nux-vomica seeds), E Zhu (zedoary rhizome, zedoaria)
C. Shui Zhi (leech), San Leng (bur-reed rhizome, scirpus)
D. Ban Mao (Cantharides, mylabris), Mang Chong (Gadfly Female)

Answer Keys: 1C. 2D. 3C. 4D. 5A. 6A. 7C. 8B. 9C. 10D

Chapter 10 Herbs that Transform Phlegm and Stop Cough

Classification:

1. Cool herbs that transform Phlegm-Heat
2. Warm herbs that transform Phlegm-Cold
3. Herbs that relieve cough and wheezing

Section 1 Herbs that Transform Phlegm-Cold

1. Ban Xia (Rhizoma Pinellae Ternatae) 半夏
2. Tian Nan Xing (Rhizoma Arisaematis) 天南星
3. Bai Jie Zi (Semen Sinapis Albae) 白芥子
4. Bai Fu Zi (Rhizoma Typhonii Gigantei) 白附子
5. Bai Qian (Radix et Rhizoma Cynanchi) 白前
6. Xuan Fu Hua (Flos Inulae) 旋覆花
7. Zao Jia (Fructus Gleditsiae) 皂荚

Name	Property	CN	Actions & Indications	Remarks
Ban Xia Rhizoma Pinellae Ternatae 半夏 Pinellia rhizome	Acrid Warm **Toxic**	LU SP ST	1. **Dries Dampness, transforms Phlegm**: For cough due to Phlegm. It is one of the important herb for treating Damp Phlegm and Cold Phlegm, especially Phlegm in Zhang Fu organs; used with Chen Pi, Fu Ling (as Er Chen Tang). 2. **Harmonizes Stomach:** for nausea, vomiting due to Stomach Qi rebelleouslly go upward. It is one of the important herbs for treating vomiting; used with Shen Jiang (as Xiao Ban Xia Tang). 3. **Dissipates nodules:** for chest distention, chest pain, plum pit.	3-10g internally. Only processed Ban Xia is used. **Incompatible with Wu Tou** Contraindication for Yin Deficiency. **More than 30g of processed Ban Xia or 0.1-2.4g unprocessed Ban Xia can be poisoning.**

			A. Epigastric and abdominal fullness or distention, used with Chen Pi, Hou Po or Gan Jiang, Huang Lian (As Ban Xia Xie Xin Tang). B. Phlegm nodules in the neck (goiter, scrofula), used with Kun Bu, Hai Zao. C. Plum pit Qi, used with Hou Po, Fu Ling (as Ban Xia Hou Po Tang). 4. **Reduces swollen and stops pain:** internally use for goiter (Ying Liu). Externally use for carbuncle, scrofula, snake bite. mixed with egg white for external use.	Based on different processing, there are different kind of Ban Xia: **Qing Ban Xia** is good at Phlegm, **Fa Ban Xia** is good at Damp Phlegm, **Jiang Ban Xia** is good at vomiting, **Zhu Li Ban Xia** is good at resolving Phlegm and distinguishes Wind, **Ban Xia Qui** is good at food stagnation.
Tian Nan Xing (Rhizoma Arisaematis) 天南星 Jack-in-the-pulpit rhizome, arisaema	Bitter Acrid Warm **Toxic**	LU SP LV	1. **Dries Dampness, transforms Phlegm:** for cough due to Damp-Cold Phlegm; used with Ban Xia, Chen Pi, Fu Ling (As Dao Tan Tang). 2. **Disperses Wind-Phlegm and stops spasm:** for dizziness, stroke, and seizure due to Wind Phlegm; used with Ban Xia, Tian Ma. 3. **Reduces swelling & stops pain:** Topically used for carbuncle, scrofula, goiter.	3-10g Toxic symptoms include burning feeling of throat, numbness of tongue and mouth, drooling, difficult to open mouth, mouth ulcer. Later on, dizziness and palpitation, numbness of limbs, coma and breathing stops. Skin contact can lead to itching and swollen.
Bai Jie Zi (Semen Sinapis	Acrid Warm	LU	1. **Warms Lung, transforms Phlegm :** for cough and wheezing, chest distention with thin Phlegm	**3-6g** Good at expel Phlegm in

Albae) 白芥子 White mustard seed			due to Cold Phlegm; used with Zi Su Zi. **2. Dissipates nodules, reduces swellingn & stop pain:** for numbness of limbs, joint pain and swollen due to Phlegm in the channels, body ache, Yin type boil due to Cold Phlegm (as in Yang He Tang). **3. External use as point plaster** in the summer to prevent cough and wheezing in winter.	channels. Large dosage internally use can cause gastrointestinal tract disorders with abdominal pain and diarrhea.
Bai Fu Zi (Rhizoma Typhonii Gigantei) 白附子 Typhonium rhizome	Sweet Acrid Warm **Toxic**	LV ST	1. **Transforms Wind-Phlegm**: for stoke, facial paralysis, headache, especially migraine. **A.** Wind stroke, facial paralysis, hemiplegia, or tetanus due to Wind Phlegm, used with Jiang Can, Quan Xie (as Qian Zheng San) for facial paralysis; used with Tian Nan Xing, Tian Ma, and Fang Feng for tetanus. B. Pain or numbness due to Cold-Phlegm or Wind-Phlegm, such as migraine headaches, used with Bai Zhi, Chuan Xiong. **2. Resolves toxicity & dissipates nodules**: for scrofula, carbuncle, snake bite; used with Xu Chang Qing for snake bite; usually used topically with Xiong Hang for scrofula and carbuncle due to Phlegm and toxicity.	**3-6g**
Bai Qian (Radix et Rhizoma Cynanchi) 白前	Acrid Sweet Slightly warm	LU	**Guides Lung Qi downward, transforms Phlegm:** for all kinds of wheezing and cough due to Lung Qi losing descending due to Phlegm obstruction.	3-10g Do not use it for dry cough. It can irritate Stomach, do not use it for

root and rhizome of cynanchum			A. Cold type: used with Ban Xia, Zi Wan. B. Heat type: used with Sang Bai Pi, Di Gu Pi. C; used with gurgling in the throat with Zi Wan, Ban Xia.	Stomach ulcer or Stomach bleeding patents.
Xuan Fu Hua (Flos Inulae) 旋覆花 Inula flower	Bitter Acrid Salty Slightly warm	LU SP ST LV	1. **Guides Lung Qi downward & transforms sputum:** for cough and wheezing with Phlegm and chest congestion; used with Ban Xia, Xi Xin. 2. **Guides Stomach Qi downward:** for vomiting, belching and hiccup; used with Ban Xia, Dai Zhe Shi (As Xuan Fu Dai Zhe Tang).	3-10g. **Wrapped.**
Zao Jia (Fructus Gleditsiae) 皂荚 Chinese honeylocust fruit, gleditsia	Acrid Salty Warm **Toxic**	LU LI	1. **Transforms sputum:** for cough; used with Da Zao, or Ban Xia, Gan Cao. 2. **Opens orifices:** for loss of consciousness. 3. **Expels Wind and kills parasites:** for dermatosis; used with Jin Yin Hua, Bai Zhi.	1.5-5g Good at expel hard Phlegm
Zao Jiao Ci 皂角刺 (Gleditsiae Spina)	Acrid Warm	LV ST LU	1. **Reduces swellings, discharges pus, invigorates Blood, reduces abscesses:** for early stages of swollen sores to encourage suppuration or to burst. 2. **Expels Wind, kills parasites:** leprosy and ringworm.	3-9g

Practice 21

1. Which of the following herbs is incompatible with Wu Tou (radix acnoite)?
A. Du Huo (Angelicae Pubescentis, Radix)
B. Ban Xia (Pinelliae Ternatae, Rhizoma)
C. Bai Fu Zi (Rhizoma Typhonii Gigantei)
D. Pi Pa Ye (Eriobotryae Japonicae, Folium)

2. Which of the following herbs needs to be wrapped for decoction?
A. Bai Qian (Radix et Rhizoma Cynanchi)
B. Sha Ren (Amonmi, Fructum)
C. Xuan Fu Hua (Inulae, Flos)
D. Ban Xia (Rhizoma Pinellae Ternatae)

3. What kind of Ban Xia (Pinelliae Ternatae, Rhizoma) should NOT be taken orally?
A. Jiang Ban Xia (prepared with alumen, fresh ginger)
B. Sheng Ban Xia (unprepared)
C. Zhi Ban Xia (prepared with alumen, fresh ginger, and lime)
D. Ban Xia Qu (fermented with flour)

4. Which of the following herbs is the best to transform Damp(Cold)-Phlegm , and descend rebellious Stomach Qi downward to stop vomiting?
A. Ban Xia (Pinelliae Ternatae, Rhizoma)
B. Xuan Fu Hua (Flos Inulae)
C. Huo Xiang (Agastaches seu Pogostemi, Herba)
D. Zhu Ru (Bambusae in Taeniis, Caulis)

5. Which of the following herbs used topically is good for asthma of Cold type, but may cause skin lesion in patients with sensitive skin?
A. Ban Xia (Rhizoma Pinellae Ternatae)
B. Bai Jie Zi (Sinapis Albae, Semen)
C. Pang Da Hai (Sterculiae Scaphigerae, Semen)
D. Zao Jia (Fructus Gleditsiae)

6. Which of the following herbs can direct both rebellious Lung and Stomach Qi downward and are good for cough, wheezing, vomiting, and hiccoughs due to Cold (Damp) Phlegm accumulation?
A. Xuan Fu Hua (Inulae, Flos)
B. Qian Hu (Peucedani, Radix)

C. Bai Fu Zi (Typhonii Gigantei, Rhizoma)
D. Huo Xiang (Agastaches seu Pogostemi, Herba)

7. Which of the following is the function of Bai Qian (Cynanchi Baiqian, Radix et Rhizoma)?
A. Dispel Wind-Dampness to relieve Bi syndrome
B. Extinguishing internal Wind and relieving spasm
C. Directing Stomach Qi downward to stop vomiting
D. Transforming Phlegm and descending adverse Lung Qi to stop cough

8. Tian Nan Xing (Arisaematis,Rhizoma) and Bai Fu Zi (Typhonii Gigantei, Rhizoma) share which of the following functions?
A. Drying Dampness and transforming Phlegm
B. Clearing Heat from the Lungs and Stomach
C. Transform Heat Phlegm
D. Moisten the Lung and large Intestine

9. Which of the following herb is the most effective in treating Damp and Phlegm?
A. Chuan Bei Mu (Bulbus Fritillariae Cirrhosae)
B. Ban Xia (Pinelliae Ternatae, Rhizoma)
C. Tian Nan Xing (Rhizoma Arisaematis)
D. Dan Nan Xing (prepared Tian Nan Xing with ox bile)

10. Which herbs are often combined with Ban Xia to treat Damp and Phlegm?
A. Cang Zhu, Bai Zhu
B. Chen Pi, Fu Ling
C. Hou Po, Sha Ren
D. Sha Ren, Yi Yi Ren

11. Which herb is effective in treating Wind-Phlegm?
A. Tian Nan Xing (Rhizoma Arisaematis)
B. Dan Nan Xing (prepared Tian Nan Xing with ox bile)
C. Bai Jie Zi (Semen Sinapis Albae)
D. All of the above

12. Which herb is best for treating aching and numbness sensation of the extremities and joints?
A. Bai Jie Zi (Semen Sinapis Albae)
B. Chuan Bei Mu (Bulbus Fritillariae Cirrhosae)

C. Xuan Fu Hua (Inulae, Flos)
D. Ban Xia (Pinelliae Ternatae, Rhizoma)

13. Which of the following herbs can strongly dispel Phlegm, open the orifices to revive the spirit and dissipate clumps, reduce swellings as well as kill parasites?
A. Xuan Fu Hua (Inulae, Flos)
B. Qian Hu (Peucedani, Radix)
C. Bai Fu Zi (Typhonii Gigantei, Rhizoma)
D. Zao Jiao (Chinese honeylocust fruit, gleditsia)

14. Which of the following herbs can be externally used as point plaster in the summer to prevent from coughing and wheezing in winter?
A. Xuan Fu Hua (Inulae, Flos)
B. Qian Hu (Peucedani, Radix)
C. Bai Fu Zi (Typhonii Gigantei, Rhizoma)
D. Bai Jie Zi (Semen Sinapis Albae)

15. What of the following statement about difference between Ban Xia (Pinelliae Ternatae, Rhizoma) and Tian Nan Xing (Rhizoma Arisaematis) is correct?
A. Ban Xia is better for Damp-Phlegm in Spleen and Lung
B. Tian Nan Xing is better for Damp-Phlegm in channels, such as dizziness, stroke, facial paralysis, tetanus due to Phlegm accumulation or Wind-Damp obstruction in channels
C. Dan Nan Xing is better in convulsion and twitch due to Heat-Phlegm than Tian Nan Xing
D. All of above

16. Diarrhea as the main complaint. There is diarrhea with borborygmus, full stuffy but painless feeling in epigastrum, dry heaves or frank vomiting, poor appetite, tongue coating thin yellow, pulse wiry. What is the diagnosis?
A. Disharmony between Stomach and Intestine
B. Damp Heat in the Middle Jiao
C. Cold in the large Intestine
D. None of them

17. What do you think treatment plans are based on question No. 16?
A. Harmonize the Stomach, direct rebellious qi downward, disperse clumping, and eliminate focal distention.
B. Clear Heat and drain Dampness
C. Dispel Cold in the large Intestine

D. None of them

18. What main herbs do you think can treat the problems based on question No. 16?
A. Ban Xia (Pinelliae Ternatae, Rhizoma)
B. Huang Lian (rhizoma coptidis chinesis)
C. Gui Zhi (radix cinnamomi cassiae)
D. None of them

Answer Keys: 1B. 2B. 3B. 4A. 5B. 6A. 7D. 8A. 9B. 10B. 11D. 12A. 13D. 14D. 15D. 16A. 17A. 18A

Section 2 Herbs that Transform Phlegm-Heat

Common characters:

1. Most of them are bitter Cold or sweet Cold and used for treating coughing caused by Phlegm-Heat or dry Phlegm.
2. Some are salty Cold herbs that can soften hardness.

Herbs:

1. Chuan Bei Mu (Bulbus Fritillariae Cirrhosae) 川贝母
2. Zhe Bei Mu (Bulbus Fritillariae Thunbergii) 浙贝母
3. Qian Hu (Radix Peucedani) 前胡
4. Gua Lou (Fractus Trichosanthis) 瓜蒌
5. Zhu Ru (Caulis Bambusae in Taeniis) 竹茹
6. Zhu Li (Succus Bambusae) 竹沥
7. Tian Zhu Huang (Concreto Silicea Bambusae) 天竺黄
8. Hai Zao (Herba Sargassii) 海藻
9. Kun Bu (Thallus Algae) 昆布
10. Meng Shi(Lapis Micae seu Chloriti) 礞石
11. Pang Da Hai (Semen Sterculiae Scsphigerae) 胖大海
12. Hai Ge Qiao/Ke (Concha Cyclinae) 海蛤壳

Name	Property	CN	Actions & Indications	Remarks
Chuan Bei Mu (Bulbus Fritillariae Cirrhosae) 川贝母 Tendrilled fritillaria bulb, fritillaria	Bitter Sweet Slightly Cold	LU HT	1. **Clears Heat and transforms Phlegm:** for cough caused by Phlegm-Heat, dry Phlegm or Yin Deficiency. A. due to Heat-Phlegm, used with Zhi Mu (Er Mu San). B. due to Wind-Heat or stagnation of Phlegm Fire, used with Sang Ye, Xing Ren. C. Chronic cough due to Lung Deficiency, used with Sha Shen, Mai Men Dong, Tian Men Dong. 2. **Clears toxicity and**	3-10g **Incompatible with Wu Tou** Good at coughing caused by Yin Deficiency.

			dissipates nodules: for Lung abscess and nodules. A. scrofula, used with Xuan Shen, Mu Li. B. Brest carbuncles, used with Pu Gong Ying, Tian Hua Fen C. Lung abscess, with Yu Xing Cao, Lu Gen, Yi Yi Ren.	
Zhe Bei Mu (Bulbus Fritillariae Thunbergii) 浙贝母 Thunberg fritillaria bulb, Fritillaria	Bitter Cold	LU HT	1. **Clears Heat and transforms Phlegm:** for coughing caused by Phlegm-Heat, dry Phlegm or Yin Deficiency. 2. **Clears toxicity and dissipates nodules:** for Lung abscess and nodules.	3-10g **Incompatible with Wu Tou** Good at clearing toxicity.
Qian Hu (Radix Peucedani) 前胡 Hogfennel root, Peucedanum	Bitter Acrid Slightly Cold	LU	1. **Guides Qi downward and expels Phlegm:** for coughing caused by Phlegm-Heat; used with Xing Ren, Sang Bai Pi, Bei Mu. 2. **Expels Wind-Heat:** for Wind Heat coughing; used with Bo He, Niu Bang Zi, Jie Geng.	6-10g
Gua Lou (Fractus Trichosanthis) 瓜蒌 Trichosanthes fruit	Sweet Cold	LI LU ST	1. **Clears Heat and transforms Phlegm:** for coughing caused by Phlegm-Heat or dry Phlegm; used with Huang Qin. 2. **Expands chest:** for chest pain. A. due to obstruction of Phlegm-Qi in chest, used with Xie Bai (as Gua Luo Xie Bai Ba Xia Tang).	10-20g **Incompatible with Wu Tou.** **Gua Lou Pi** (peel of Gua Lou) is good at expanding chest, **Gua Lou Ren** is good at lubricating

			B. due to accumulation of Heat-Phlegm, used with Ban Xia, Huang Lian (as Xiao Xian Xiong Tang). 3. **Expends chest, dissipate abscess:** for Lung, Intestine and breast abscesses; used with Pu Gong Ying, JinYin Hua; Yu Xing Cao. 4. **Lubricates Intestine:** for constipation; used with Huo Ma Ren.	Intestine
Zhu Ru (Caulis Bambusae in Taeniis) 竹茹 Bamboo shavings	Sweet Slightly Cold	GB LU ST	1. **Clears Heat and transforms Phlegm:** for coughing caused by Phlegm-Heat; used with Huang Qin, Gua Lou. 2. **Clams Shen:** for insomnia caused by coughing or caused by Phlegm-Fire disturbing Heart; used with Chen Pi, Fu Ling, Zhi Shi (Wen Dan Tang). 3. **Stops vomiting:** for Stomach Heat vomiting; used with Chen Pi (as Ju Pi Zhu Ru Tang) 4. **Cools Blood:** for bleeding due to Blood Heat.	6-10g Contraindication for Stomach and Spleen Yang Deficiency or Cold food stagnation.
Zhu Li (Succus Bambusae) 竹沥 Dried bamboo sap	Sweet **Very Cold**	HT LU ST	1. **Clears Heat and transforms Phlegm:** for coughing caused by Phlegm-Heat; used with Jiang Ban Xia, Huang Qin 2. **Opens orifices:** for stroke and epilepsy; used alone or with Sheng Jiang juice.	**15-30ml**
Tian Zhu Huang (Concreto	Sweet Cold	GB HT	1. **Clears Heat and transforms Phlegm:** for coughing caused by Phlegm-Heat.	**3-6g**

Silicea Bambusae) 天竺黄 Siliceous Secretions of Bamboo		LR	2. **Clears Heart and stops convulsion:** for convulsion.	
Hai Zao (Herba Sargassii) 海藻 Seaweed, Sargassum	Bitter Salty Cold	KI LR ST LU	1. **Resolves Phlegm and softens hardness:** for goiter; used with Jiang Can, Xia Ku Cao. 2. **Promotes urination:** for edema.	10-15g. Incompatible with **Gan Cao** Iodine is inside.
Kun Bu (Thallus Algae) 昆布 Kelp thallus, Laminaria	Salty Cold	KI LR ST	1. **Reduces Phlegm and softens hardness:** for goiter; used with Hai Zao (as Kun Bu Wan). 2. **Promotes urination:** for edema.	6-12g Iodine is inside.
Pang Da Hai (Semen Sterculiae Scsphigerae) 胖大海 Boat sterculia seed	Sweet Cold	LI LU	1. **Clears Heat and benefits throat:** Sore throat, hoarseness, use alone or with Jie Geng, Niu Bang Zi. 2. **Clears Lung Heat and moves bowels:** Cough due to Heat-Phlegm, use alone or with Jie Geng, Chan Tui, Bo He. For constipation due to Heat, use alone.	2-4 pieces
Meng Shi (Lapis Micae seu Chloriti) 礞石 Lapis Stone	Sweet, Salty neutral	LI LV	1. **Resolves Phlegm:** for coughing and wheezing due to hard to treat Phlegm. 2. **Calms Liver:** for mania, convulsion due to Phlegm.	5-10g. Decoct early and wrapped. Contraindication for pregnancy
Hai Ge Qiao/Ke (Concha Cyclinae)	Bitter Salty	KI LU	1. **Clears Lung Heat and transforms Phlegm:** for cough.	10-15g Decoct early

海蛤壳 Cyclina	Neutral	ST	2. **Softens hardness and dissipates nodules:** for goiter, scrofula	
Hou Zao (Calculus Macacae Mulattae) 猴枣 Macaque Bezoar	Bitter Salty Cold	GB HT LR LU	1. **dislodges Phlegm and controls spasm** 2. **Arrests wheezing**	
Ze Qi (Herba Euphorbiae Helioscopiae) 泽漆 Euphorbia	Acrid Bitter Cool **Slightly toxic**	SI LI LU	1. **Transforms Phlegm and controls spasm** 2. **Dissipates nodules** 3. **promotes urination**	
HUANG YAO ZI (Tuber Dioscoreae Bulbiferae) 黄药子 Dioscorea Bulbifera Tuber	Bitter Neutral **Toxic**	HT LRL U	1. **Reduces Phlegm and softens hardness:** for goiter 2. **Clears Heat and reduces toxicity:** for carbuncle, swollen throat and snake bite 3. **Cools Blood and stops bleeding:** for bleeding	5-15g

Practice 22

1. Which of the following is an indication of Qian Hu (Peucedani, Radix)?
A. Bi Syndrome due to Wind-Heat-Dampness
B. Dampness in the Middle Jiao
C. Cough due to Wind Heat
D. Restless fetus due to Liver and Kidney Deficiency

2. What is the difference between Chuan Bei Mu (Fritillariae Carrhosae, Bulbus) and Zhe Bei Mu (Fritillariae Thunbergii, Bulbus)?
A. Chuan Bei Mu is Cold in property, Zhe Bei Mu is warm in property
B. Chuan Bei Mu is stronger at moistening Lung, Zhe Bei Mu is stronger at clearing Heat and dissipating nodules
C. Chuan Bei Mu is incompatible with Wu Tou (radix aconite), Zhe Bei Mu is incompatible with Gan Cao (licorice root)
D. All of the above

3. Which of the following herbs has the functions of resolving Phlegm and promoting the flow of Qi to relieve chest oppression, and is commonly used for chest Bi?
A. Tian Nan Xing (arisaema)
B. Gua Lou (Trichosanthis, Fructus)
C. Xu Duan (Dipsaci Asperi, Radix)
D. Sha Ren (Amonmi, Fructum)

4. Which of the following herbs is the best for vomiting due to Stomach Heat?
A. Huo Xiang (Agastaches seu Pogostemi, Herba)
B. Ban Xia (Pinelliae Ternatae, Rhizoma)
C. Xuan Fu Hua (Inulae, Flos)
D.Zhu Ru (Bambusae in Taeniis, Caulis)

5. Which of the following herbs can be used as tea (infusion) for benefiting throat and improving voice?
A. Pang Da Hai (Sterculiae Scaphigerae, Semen)
B. Qian Hu (Peucedani, Radix)
C. Gua Lou (Trichosanthis, Fructus)
D. Zhu Ru (Bambusae in Taeniis, Caulis)

6. Which of the following herb groups is the best for goiter and scrofula due to

Phlegm?
A. Bai Dou Kou (Amomi Kravanh, Fructus), Sha Ren (Amonmi, Fructum)
B. Kun Bu (Algae, Thallus), Hai Zao (Sargassii, Herba)
C. Xu Duan (Dipsaci Asperi, Radix), Sang Ji Sheng (Taxilus chinensis (DC.) Danser)
D. Zhu Ru (Bambusae in Taeniis, Caulis), Gua Lou (Trichosanthis, Fructus)

7. Which of the following herbs is best for cough due to LU yin Deficiency?
A. Chuan Bei Mu (Fritillariae Carrhosae, Bulbus)
B. Zhe Bei Mu (Fritillariae Thunbergii, Bulbus)
C. Ban Xia (Pinellia Rhizome)
D. Ma Huang (Ephedra)

8. Which herb is incompatible with Hai Zao?
A. Kun Bu (Algae, Thallus)
B. Sheng Jiang (Fresh Ginger)
C. Da Zao (Dry Date)
D. Gan Cao (Licorice root)

9. Which herb is incompatible with Wu Tou?
A. Chuan Bei Mu (Fritillariae Carrhosae, Bulbus)
B. Gua Lou (Trichosanthis, Fructus)
C. Zhe Bei Mu (Fritillariae Thunbergii, Bulbus)
D. All of the above

10. Which herb not only descends LU Qi, expel Phlegm, but also dispel Exterior Wind-Heat?
A. Qian Hu (Peucedani, Radix)
B. Chuan Bei Mu (Fritillariae Carrhosae, Bulbus)
C. Zhe Bei Mu (Fritillariae Thunbergii, Bulbus)
D. Gua Lou (Trichosanthis, Fructus)

11. The qi of Jie Geng (Radix Platycodi Grandiflori) is:
A. Upbearing
B. Downbearing
C. Entering
D. Out-thrusting

12. Which of the following herbs is incompatible with Gan Cao (licorice root)?
A. Ban Xia (Pinelliae Ternatae, Rhizoma)
B. Jie Geng (Radix Platycodi Grandiflori)

C. Pa Da Hai (Sterculiae Scaphigerae, Semen)
D. Hai Zao (Sargassii, Herba)

13. Which of the following herbs is the best for cough with thick, yellow sputum, a red tongue with yellow, greasy coating, and a slippery, rapid pulse?
A. Tian Nan Xing (arisaema)
B. Gua Lou (Trichosanthis, Fructus)
C. Cao Dou Kou (Alpiniae Katsumadai, Semen)
D. Bai Fu Zi (Typhonii Gigantei, Rhizoma

Answer Keys: 1C. 2B. 3B. 4D. 5A. 6B. 7A. 8D. 9D. 10A. 11A. 12D. 13B

Section 3 Herbs that Stop Cough and Wheezing

1. (Ku) Xing Ren (Semen Pruni Armeniacae) 杏仁
2. Bai Bu (Radix Stemonae) 百部
3. Su Zi (Fructus Perileae Frutescentis) 苏子
4. Jie Geng (Radis Platycodi Grandiflori) 桔梗
5. Zi Wan (Radix Asteris Tatarici) 紫菀
6. Kuan Dong Hua (Flos Tussilaginis Farfarae) 款冬花
7. Sang Bai Pi (Cotex Mori Albae Radicis) 桑白皮
8. Pi Pa Ye (Folium Eriobotryae) 枇杷叶
9. Ting Li Zi (Semen Descurainiae seu Lepiddi) 葶苈子

Name	Property	CN	Actions & Indications	Remarks
Xing Ren / Ku Xing Ren (Semen Pruni Armeniacae) 杏仁 Apricot seed or kernel	Bitter, slightly warm, **slightly toxic**	LU LI	1. **Stops cough, calms wheezing:** for cough & wheezing. A. Cool Dryness, used with Zi SuYe, Chen Pi, Qian Hu (as Xing Su San). B. Wind Heat, used with Sang Ye, Ju Hua (as Sang Ju Yin). C. Warm Dryness, used with Sang Ye, Bei Mu (Sang Xing Tang). D. Excessive Heat in the Lung, used with Shi Gao, Ma Huang (as Ma Xing Shi Gan Tang). **2. Moistens Intestine & moves bowels:** for constipation, used with Huo Ma Ren, Bai Shao.	5-10g. Smashed before decocting. Use with caution for children. Contraindicate with Yin Deficiency and loose stool. Use with caution for infants. 30g or more can be poisoning.
Bai Bu (Radix Stemonae) 百部 Stemona root	Sweet, bitter, slightly warm	LU	**1. Moistens Lung, stops cough:** for cough and wheezing. A. Due to external Wind-Cold, used with Ma Huang, Xing Ren. B. Due to Wind, used with Jing	5-15g 30-60g for treating pinworm.

			Jie, Jie Geng (as Zhi Su San). C. Due to Lung Yin Deficiency, used with Mai Men Dong, Sheng Di Huang, Chuan Bei Mu. D. Due to Lung Heat, used with Bei Mu, Zi Wan. **2. Expels parasites, kills lice:** for pinworm/threadworm, trichomonad, lice and parasitic mite (Sarcoptes scabiei); used with Ku Shen (as external wash).	
Su Zi (Fructus Perileae Frutescentis) 苏子 Purple perilla fruit, Perilla seed	Acrid, warm	LU LI	**1. Guides Lung Qi downward:** for cough and wheezing due to Phlegm; used with Bai Jie, Lai Fu Zi (as San Zi Yang Qin Tang). **2. Moistens Intestine:** for constipation; used with Huo Ma Ren, Gua Lou Ren, Xing Ren.	5-10g
Jie Geng (Radis Platycodi Grandiflori) 桔梗 Balloon Flower Rhizome	Bitter, acrid, neutral	LU	**1. Disseminates Lung Qi, resolves Phlegm:** for cough. A. due to Wind-Heat, used with Sang Ye, Ju Hua, Xing Ren (as Sang Ju Yin). B. due to Wind-Cold, used with Xing Ren, Su Ye (as Xing Su San). **2. Discharges pus:** for Lung abscess; used with Gan Cao; or Lu Gen, Yi Yi Ren, Yu Xing Cao. **3. Benefits throat:** for sore throat; used with Bo He, Niu Bang Zi, Chan Tui.	3-10g Over dosage will cause vomiting. Contraindicated with vomiting, hemoptysis.

Zi Wan (Radix Asteris Tatarici) 紫菀 Purple aster root, Aster	Bitter, slightly warm	LU	**1.Moistens Lung, resolves Phlegm and stops cough:** for cough and wheezing due to any reason. A. Cough with profuse Phlegm due to Phlegm stagnation, used with Kuan Dong Hua. B. Cough with profuse sputum due to external Wind Cold, used with Jing Jie, Bai Qian, Chen Pi. C. Cough with Blood due to Lung Deficiency, used with Zhi Mu, Bei Mu, Er Jiao.	5-10g Comparison with Kuan Dong Hua, it is good at resolving Phlegm. Can be used for all kind of cough.
Kuan Dong Hua (Flos Tussilaginis Farfarae) 款冬花 Coltsfoot flower, Tussilago	acrid, warm	LU	**1.Moistens Lung, descends Lung Qi, resolves Phlegm and stops cough:** for cough and wheezing due to any reason. A. Due to Cold-Phlegm, used with Xi Xin, Zi Wan (She Gan Ma Huang Tang). B. Chronic cough with Blood, used with Bai He.	5-10g Comparison with Zi Wan, it is good at stopping cough. Good at Cold cough.
Sang Bai Pi (Cotex Mori Albae Radicis) 桑白皮 Bark of mulberry root, Morus bark	Sweet, Cold	LI SP	**1. Clears Lung Heat, stops cough and wheezing:** for coughg and wheezing; used with Di Gu Pi, Gan Cao (as Xie Bai San). **2. Promotes urination:** for edema due to Lung Qi dose not disperse; used with Fu Ling Pi, Da Fu Pi (as Wu Pi Yin).	5-15g; Honey fried for coughing and wheezing
Pi Pa Ye (Folium Eriobotryae) 枇杷叶 Loquat leaf, eriobotrya	Bitter, cool	LU ST	**1. Stops cough, expels Phlegm:** for cough and wheezing; used with Xing Ren, Sang Ye, Qian Hu. **2. Harmonizes Stomach:** for nausea, vomiting, hiccough; used with Xiang Fu, Bai Mao	10-15g; **Wrapped;** honey processed for cough, ginger processed juice for

			Gen.	nausea and vomiting
Ting Li Zi (Semen Descurainiae seu Lepiddi) 葶苈子 Descurainia seeds, lepidium seeds	acrid, bitter, Cold	LU BL	**1. Drains Lung, calms wheezing:** for cough and wheezing; used with Da Zao (as Ting Li Da Zao Xie Fei Tang). **2. Reduces edema**; used with Fang Ji, Da Huang (as Ji Jiao Li Huang Wan).	5-10g; 1. Contraindi-cated for cough and wheezing due to Lung Qi Deficiency. 2. Contraindi-cated for edema due to Spleen Deficiency.

Practice 23

1. Which herb can moisten the Intestines?
A. Xing Ren (Semen Pruni Armeniacae)
B. Su Zi (Fructus Perileae Frutescentis)
C. Gua Lou Ren (Fractus Trichosanthis Kernel)
D. All of the above

2. Which herb must be used cautiously for infants?
A. Xing Ren (Semen Pruni Armeniacae)
B. Zi Su Ye (Folium et Caulis Perillae)
C. Huo Xiang (Herba Pogostemonis)
D. Gan Cao (Radix Glycyrrhizae)

3. Su Zi (Fructus Perileae Frutescentis) is used for
A. Cough with copious Phlegm
B. Stiffling sensation in the chest
C. Constipation
D. All of the above

4. What is the common function of Zi Wan (Asteris Tatarici, Radix) and Kuan Dong Hua (Tussilaginis Farfarae, Flos)?
A. Clear LU, stop cough, expel Phlegm
B. Moisten LU, stop cough, expel Phlegm
C. Astringe LU, stop cough, expel Phlegm
D. Purge LU, stop cough, expel Phlegm

5. Common function of Zhu Ru (Caulis Bambusae in Taeniis) and Pi Pa Ye (Eriobotryae Japonicae, Folium) is
A. Descend ST Qi and stop vomiting
B. Clear Heat and remove irritability
C. Kill parasites and stop itching
D. Moisten Intestines

6. Which herb lubricates the LU, stops cough and kills parasites and worms?
A. Zi Wan (Asteris Tatarici, Radix)
B. Kuan Dong Hua (Tussilaginis Farfarae, Flos)
C. Xing Ren (Semen Pruni Armeniacae)
D. Bai Bu (Radix Stemonae)

7. Which herb is warm and moistening, but is not dry or greasy and can stop coughing

and asthma?
A. Zi Wan (Asteris Tatarici, Radix)
B. Kuan Dong Hua (Tussilaginis Farfarae, Flos)
C. Bai Bu (Radix Stemonae)
D. All of the above

8. Which of the following herbs is most effective in purging LU Heat and calming asthma?
A. Shi Gao (Gypsum fibrous)
B. Zhi Mu (Rhizoma Anemarrhenae)
C. Sang Bai Pi (Cotex Mori Albae Radicis)
D. Huang Qin (Radix Scutellariae)

9. What is the common channel of “Transforming Phlegm” and “Stop cough” category herbs?
A. LU
B. SP
C. KD
D. LV

10. If a patient complains of edema with urinary difficulty, accompanied by cough, wheezing, fullness in the chest, red tongue with yellow coating, slippery and rapid pulse, which of the following herbs is the best?
A. Kuan Dong Hua (Tussilaginis Farfarae, Flos)
B. Zi Wan (Asteris Tatarici, Radix)
C. Pi Pa Ye (Eriobotryae Japonicae, Folium)
D. Ting Li Zi (Descurainiae seu Lepidii, Semen)

11. Which of the following herbs is the best for sore throat, hoarseness and loss of voice due to Wind Heat attacking the Lungs?
A. Sang Bai pi ((Mori Albae Radicis, Cortex)
B. Mu Hu Die(Oroxyli Indici, Semen)
C. Kuan Dong Hua (Tussilaginis Farfarae, Flos)
D. Zi Wan (Asteris Tatarici, Radix)

12. What is the difference between Kuan Dong Hua (Tussilaginis Farfarae, Flos) and Zi Wan (Asteris Tatarici, Radix)?
A. Kuan Dong Hua can direct Stomach Qi downward to stop vomiting, Zi Wan cannot
B. Zi Wan can moisten Lung, Kuan Dong Hua cannot
C. Kuan Dong Hua is better at descending rebellious Lung Qi
D. Zi Wan is better at descending rebellious Lung Qi

13. Which of the following herbs can stop cough due to Lung Heat?
A. Pi Pa Ye (Folium Eriobotryae)
B. Sang Bai Pi (Cotex Mori Albae Radicis)
C. Luo Han Guo (Fractus Momordicae)
D. All of above

14. Which of the following herbs can direct the effect of other herbs upward to upper region of body?
A. Bai Dou Kou (Amomi Kravanh, Fructus)
B. Hou Po (Magnoliae Officinalis, Cortex)
C. Jie Geng (Platycodi Granorum, Radix)
D. Sha Ren (Amonmi, Fructum)

Answer Keys: 1D. 2A. 3D. 4B. 5A. 6D. 7D. 8C. 9A. 10D. 11B. 12C. 13D. 14C

Chapter 11 Herbs that Relieve Food Stagnation

1. Shan Zha (Fructus Crataegi) 山楂
2. Shen Qu (Massa Fermentata) 神曲
3. Mai Ya (Fructus Hordei Vulgaris) 麦芽
4. Gu Ya (Fructus Oryzea Sativae) 谷芽
5. Lai Fu Zi (Semen Raphani Sativi) 莱菔子
6. Ji Nei Jin (Endothelium Corneum) 鸡内金

Name	Property	CN	Actions & Indications	Remarks
Shan Zha (Fructus Crataegi) 山楂 Hawthorn fruit	Sour sweet slightly warm	LV ST SP	1. **Improves digestion, removes food stagnation:** for abdominal distention, fullness and pain. It is good at greasy and meat stagnation; used with Shen Qu, Lai Fu Zi (as Bao He Wan). 2. **Moves Qi and Blood:** for chest pain, post partum abdominal pain, dysmenorrhea and amenorrhea. Now it is used for treating hypertension, coronary Heart disease, and hypercholesterolemia; used with brown sugar or Dang Gui, Chuan Xiong, Yi Mu Cao. 3. **Stops diarrhea:** for diarrhea due to food stagnation, Spleen Deficiency or Damp-Heat; used with Mu Xiang, Rou Dou Kou, Bian Dou.	10-15g; Use raw Shan Zha for Blood stasis, and dry-fried Shan Zha for food stagnation Recently used for treating hypertension, coronary artery disease, Used with Jue Ming Zi, Dan Shen.
Shen Qu (Massa Fermentata)	Sweet acrid warm	ST SP	1. **Improves digestion and harmonizes Stomach:** for abdominal distention, fullness and	6-15g Use with caution during

神曲 Massa fermentation			pain, borborygmus, lack of appetite, diarrhea; used with Shan Zha, Lai Fu Zi (as Bao He Wan).	pregnancy.
Mai Ya (Fructus Hordei Germinatus) 麦芽 (Barley Sprout)	Sweet neutral	LV ST SP	1. **Improves digestion and harmonizes Stomach:** for abdominal distention, fullness and pain. It is good at starch stagnation. A. Accumulation of undigested starchy food, used with Shan Zha, Shen Qu. B. Indigestion of milk in infant, Used alone. C. Indigestion due to Deficiency of Spleen and Stomach, used with Dang Shen, Fu Ling, Shan Yao. 2. **Stops lactation:** for stopping lactation. It is usually used up to 60-120g for stopping lactation. 3. **Soothes Liver Qi**: for Liver Qi stagnation as an assistant herb in formula, used with Bai Zhu, Chai Hu.	10-15g, Contraindicated in nursing mother.
Gu Ya (Fructus Sativae Germinatus) 谷芽 Sprout oryza Sprout setaria	Sweet neutral	ST SP	1. **Improves digestion and harmonizes Stomach:** for abdominal distention, fullness and pain; used with Sha Ren, Zhi Gan Cao. Weak digestion and loss of appetite associated with Spleen Deficiency, used with Bai Zhu.	9-15g
Lai Fu Zi (Semen Raphani Sativi) 莱菔子 Radish seed Raphanus	Sweet acrid neutral	LU ST SP	1. **Removes food stagnation:** for abdominal distention, fullness and pain; used with Shan Zha, Shen Qu, Chen Pi (as Bao He Wan). 2. **Descends Qi and expels Phlegm:** for cough and wheezing due to Phlegm; used	3-10g Do not use it with Ren Shen.

			alone or with Bai Jie Zi, Su Zi (as San Zi Yang Qin Tang).	
Ji Nei Jin (Endothelium Corneum) 鸡内金 Chicken gizzard	Sweet neutral	BL SI ST SP	1. **Improves digestion and strengthens Stomach:** for food stagnation. A. Abdominal distention, Used alone or with Shan Zha, Shen Qu, Mai Ya. B. Abdominal distention with Spleen Deficiency, used with Bai Zhu, Shan Yao, Fu Ling. 2. **Stablizes essence and stops enuresis:** for spermatorrhea and enuresis; used with Sang Piao Xiao, Fu Pen Zi. 3. **Dissolves stone:** for Kidney, gallbladder stone; used with Jin Qian Cao, Hai Jin Sha.	3-10g Powder 1.5-3g Powder is better

Practice 24

1. Which digestive herb is especially for indigestion for meaty foods?
A. Shan Zha (hawthorn fruit)
B. Ma Ya (barley sprout)
C. Ji Nei Jin (chicken gizzard's internal lining)
D. Lai Fu Zi (radish seed)

2. Which herb can activate the Blood and removes stasis?
A. Mai Ya (barley sprout)
B. Gu Ya (rice sprout)
C. Shen Qu (medicated leaven)
D. Shan Zha (hawthorn fruit)

3. Which digestive herb enters the LV channel and soothes the LV Qi when it is used raw?
A. Shan Zha (hawthorn fruit)
B. Mai Ya (barley sprout)
C. Gu Ya (rice sprout)
D. Lai Fu Zi (radish seed)

4. Large dosage of stir-fried Mai Ya (barley sprout) can
A. Quiet the fetus
B. Hasten birth
C. Promote lactation
D. Inhibit lactation

5. Which herb can be added to pills containing heavy minerals to aid in digestion and absorption?
A. Shan Zha (hawthorn fruit)
B. Shen Qu (medicated leaven)
C. Ji Nei Jin (chicken gizzard's internal lining)
D. Lai Fu Zi (radish seed)

6. Ji Nei Jin (chicken gizzard's internal lining) can be used for the treatment of___
A. Constipation
B. Diarrhea
C. Promote lactation
D. Billiary tract stones

7. Which digestive herb is often taken as powder or pill in order to gain more effects?
A. Shen Qu (medicated leaven)
B. Lai Fu Zi (radish seed)
C. Mai Ya (barley sprout)
D. Lai Fu Zi (radish seed)

8. Which digestive herb can descend Qi and transform Phlegm?
A. Shan Zha (hawthorn fruit)
B. Ji Nei Jin (chicken gizzard's internal lining)
C. Shen Qu (medicated leaven)
D. Lai Fu Zi (radish seed)

9. Which of the following herbs should not use when taking Lai Fu Zi (radish seed)?
A. Ren Shen (Ginseng)
B. Ji Nei Jin (chicken gizzard's internal lining)
C. Shen Qu (medicated leaven)
D. Lai Fu Zi (radish seed)

10. Which of the following herbs is good for starchy food stagnation?
A. Shen Qu (medicated leaven)
B. Ji Nei Jin (chicken gizzard's internal lining)
C. Mai Ya (barley sprout)
D. Lai Fu Zi (radish seed)

11. Which of the following herbs can secure essence and use for frequent urination?
A. Shan Zha (hawthorn fruit)
B. Shen Qu (medicated leaven)
C. Ji Nei Jin (chicken gizzard's internal lining)
D. Lai Fu Zi (radish seed)

Answer Keys: 1A. 2D. 3B. 4D. 5B. 6D. 7A. 8D. 9A. 10C. 11C

Chapter 12 Herbs that Warm the Interior and Expel Cold

Common characters:

1. Hot or warm.
2. Enter SP, ST, KI, HT and LV, LU channels

Contraindications:

1. Excess Heat
2. False Cold with true Heat
3. Yin Deficiency Heat
4. Blood and body fluid Deficiency
5. Use with caution for pregnant women and hot season

Herbs:

1. Fu Zi (Radix Aconiti Lateralis Praeparata) 附子
2. Gan Jiang (Rhizoma Zingiberis) 干姜
3. Rou Gui (Cortex Cinnamomi) 肉桂
4. Xiao Hui Xiang (Fructus Foenicuii) 小茴香
5. Wu Zhu Yu (Fructus Evodiae) 吴茱萸
6. Ding Xiang (Flos Caryophylli) 丁香
7. Hua Jiao (Pericarpium Zanthoxyli) 花椒
8. Gao Liang Jiang (Rhizoma Alpiniae Officinarum) 高良姜
9. Hu Jiao (Fructus Piperis) 胡椒

Name	Property	CN	Actions & Indications	Remarks
Fu Zi (Radix Aconiti Lateralis Praeparata) 附子 Aconite	Acrid Sweet **Very hot and very Toxic**	HT KI SP	1. **Rescues collapsed Yang:** for Cold extremities with Cold sweating, very weak pulse due toYang collapse It is one of the important herbs for treating Yang collapse; used with Gan jiang (As Si Ni Tang). 2. **Ignites Fire to assist Yang:** for Cold extremities, soreness of lower back	3-15g. **60 minutes more decoction than other herbs to reduce its toxicity. Incompatible with Bei Mu,**

			and knee, impotence, infertility, frequent urination due to Kidney Yang Deficiency; abdominal Cold pain, diarrhea due to Spleen Yang Deficiency; edema due to Kidney and Spleen Yang Deficiency; Heart pain, palpitation, shortness of breath due to Heart Yang Deficiency; Yin type jaundice due to Spleen Yang Deficiency. A. Kidney Yang Deficiency, used with Rou Gui, Shu Di, Shan Yu Ruo (as Shen Qi Wan). B. Spleen Yang Deficiency, Used with Ren Shen, Gan Jiang , Bai Zhu, Gan Cao (as fu Zi Li Zhong Wan). C. Heart Yang Deficiency, used with Ren Shen, Gui Zhi, Gan Cao. D. Both Spleen Yang and Kidney Yang Deficiency, used with Bai Zhu , Fu Ling, Shen Jiang (as Zhen Wu Tang). 3. **Disperses Cold and alleviates pain:** for Damp-Cold Bi syndrome, used with Gui Zhi, Bai Zhu, Gan Cao (as Gan Cao Fu Zi Tang).	**Gua lou, Ban Xia, Ba Lian, Ba Ji. Antagonistic with Xi Jiao (Cornu Rhinoceri). It is contraindicated during pregnancy, false Cold with true Heat, and Yin Deficiency.** **Toxic side effects include arrythmia, low BP, low body tempreture and numbness of the mouth.**
Gan Jiang (Rhizoma Zingiberis) 干姜 Ginger - Dried	Acrid hot	HT LU SP ST	4. **Warms Middle Jiao and expels Cold:** for Cold abdominal pain, vomiting due to Stomach and Spleen Cold, both excess and Deficiency; used with Ren Shen, Gan Cao, Bai Zhu (as Li Zhong Wan). 5. **Rescues collapsed Yang and expels interior Cold:** for Cold extremities with Cold sweating, very weak pulse due to Yang exhaustion; used with Fu Zi, Gan Cao (as Si Ni Tang).	3-10g

			6. **Warms Lung and transforms Phlegm:** for coughing and wheezing with Cold back and clear Phlegm due to Lung Cold; used with Ma Huang, Xi Xin, Wu Wei Zi, Ban Xia (as Xiao Qing Long Tang).	
Rou Gui (Cortex Cinnamomi) 肉桂 Cassia Bark	Acrid hot sweet	HT KI LR SP	7. **Ignites Fire to assists Yang:** for Cold extremity, soreness of lower back and knee, impotence, infertility, frequent urination due to Kidney Yang Deficiency; used with Fu Zi, Shu Di, Shan Yao (as Shen Qi Wan). 8. **Disperses Cold and stops pain:** for Cold abdominal pain, vomiting, diarrhea due to Spleen and Stomach Cold; diarrhea, Cold extremity due to Spleen and Kidney Yang Deficiency; Damp-Cold Bi syndrome; chest pain due to Heart Yang Deficiency; Yin type abscesses; used with Fu Zi, Gan Jiang, Bai Zhu (as Gui Fu Li Zhong Wan). 9. **Warms and unblocks channels:** for dysmenorrhea, amenorrhea due to Chong and Ren Deficiency Cold leading to Blood stasis; used with Xiao Hui Xiang, Gan Jiang. 10. Put in Qi and Blood formulas to encourage Yang Qi for generating Qi and Blood.	**2-5g** **Antagonistic with Chi Shi Zhi** (Halloysitum rubrum).
Xiao Hui Xiang (Fructus Foenicuii) 小茴香 Fennel Seed	Acrid warm	KI LR SP ST	1. **Disperses Cold and stops pain:** for Cold hernial pain, lower abdominal pain, and dysmenorrhea; used with Rou Gui, Chen Xiang, Wu Yao (as Nuan Gan Jiang). 2. **Regulates Qi and harmonizes Stomach:** for abdominal pain, reduced appetite, vomiting; used	3-9g

			with Gan Jiang, Mu Xiang.	
Wu Zhu Yu (Fructus Evodiae) 吴茱萸 Evodia Fruit	Acrid bitter hot **slightly toxic**	KI LR SP ST	1. **Disperses Cold and stops pain:** for Cold hernial pain caused by Liver channel constraint; used with Wu Yao, Xiao Hui Xiang. 2. Jueyin headache, dysmenorrhea, abdominal pain and edema due to Cold-Dampness. A. Gastric and abdominal Cold pain, Used with Gan Jiang , Mu Xiang. B. Headache, drooling and reduced taste sensation due to deficient Cold in the Middle Jiao and rebellious Liver Qi, Used with Ren Shen, Sheng Jiang (as Wu Zhu Yu Tang). C. Irregular menstruation and dysmenorrhea, Used with Dang Gui, Chuan Xiong, E Jiao (as Wen Jing Tang). 2. **Decsends rebellious Liver Qi:** for vomiting due to Liver Fire attacking Stomach or Liver-Stomach disharmony; used with Huang Lian, (Zuo Jin Wan). 3. **Warms Yang and stops diarrhea:** for daybreak diarrhea due to Spleen and Kidney Yang Deficiency; used with Bu Gu Zhi, Rou Dou Kou (as Si Shen Wan).	**1.5-6g** Can not be used with higher dosage or long term.
Ding Xiang (Flos Caryophylli) 丁香 Clove Flower Bud	Acrid warm	KI SP ST	1. **Warms the middle and descends rebellious Qi:** for hiccup, vomiting due to Stomach Cold; used with Shu Di, Ren Shen, Sheng Jiang (as Ding Xiang Shu Di Tang). 2. **Disperses Cold and stops pain:** for Cold Stomachache and abdominal	**3-6g** **Antagonistic with Yu Jin (Tuber curcumae)**

			pain; used with Sha Ren, Bai Zhu (as Ding Xiang San). 3. **Warms Kidney Yang:** for impotence with lower back and knee soreness; used with Fu Zi, Rou Gui, Ba Ji Tian, Rou Cong Rong.	
Hua Jiao (Pericarpium Zanthoxyli) 花椒 Pepper Prickly Ash Fruit	Acrid hot **slightly toxic**	KI SP ST	1. **Warms the middle and stops pain:** for Cold Stomachache, vomiting due to Spleen and Stomach Cold. 2. **Kills parasite:** for eczema, genital itching, and roundworm.	**2-5g**
Gao Liang Jiang (Rhizoma Alpiniae Officinarum) 高良姜 Galangal Rhizome	Acrid Hot	SP ST	1. **Disperses Cold and stops pain:** for epigastric and abdominal pain, hiccup due to Spleen and Stomach Cold. 2. **Warms the middle and stops vomiting:** for vomiting due to Stomach Cold.	3-10g
Hu Jiao (Fructus Piperis) 胡椒 Pepper Fruit	Acrid hot	LI ST	1. **Warms the middle and stops pain:** for vomiting, diarrhea and abdominal pain due to Spleen and Stomach Cold. A. Epigastric and abdominal pain, diarrhea, used with Xiang Fu (as Liang Fu Wan). B. Vomiting, hiccough, used with Ban Xia, Sheng Jiang. 2. **Descends Qi and resolves Phlegm:** for epilepsy due to Qi and Phlegm covering clear orifice.	**2-4g**

Practice 25

1. Which of the following herbs should be decocted 30 minutes more than others?
A. Rou Gui
B. Fu Zi
C. Wu Zhu Yu
D. Ding Xiang

2. Which of the following herbs can stop diarrhea?
A. Xiao Hui Xiang
B. Rou Gui
C. Wu Zhu Yu
D. Ding Xiang

3. Which of the following herbs can subdue rebellious Qi for hiccough and vomiting?
A. Xiao Hui Xiang
B. Rou Gui
C. Ding Xiang
D. Gan Jiang

4. Which of the following herbs is usually used with Fu Zi?
A. Xiao Hui Xiang
B. Gan Jiang
C. Rou Gui
D. Ding Xiang

5. Which of the following herbs is the best for collapsed Yang?
A. Rou Gui
B. Fu Zi
C. Wu Zhu Yu
D. Ding Xiang

6. Which of the following herbs can kill parasite?
A. Fu Zi
B. Wu Zhu Yu
C. Ding Xiang
D. Hua Jiao

7. Which of the following herbs can NOT be used with Yu Jin?
A. Xiao Hui Xiang
B. Gan Jiang
C. Rou Gui
D. Ding Xiang

8. Which of the following herbs can NOT be used with Chi Shi Zhi?
A. Rou Gui
B. Fu Zi
C. Wu Zhu Yu
D. Ding Xiang

9. Which of the following herbs warming the interior is NOT toxic?
A. Xiao Hui Xiang
B. Fu Zi
C. Wu Zhu Yu
D. Hua Jao

Answer Keys: 1B. 2C. 3C. 4B. 5B. 6D. 7D. 8A. 9A

Chapter 13 Herbs that Calm Spirit (Shen)

Classification

1. Herbs that heavily calm spirit (Shen)
2. Nourish Heart and calm spirit (Shen)

Common characteristics:

1. They are minerals or shells.
2. They may injury Stomach Qi resulting in indigestion and loss of appetite.
3. Some of them such as Zhu Sha are toxic and should not be taken long term.

Section 1 Herbs that Heavily Calm Spirit (Shen)

1. Ci Shi (Magnetitum) 磁石
2. Hu Po (Succinum) 琥珀
3. Long Gu (Os Draconis) 龙骨
4. Zhen Zhu (Margarita) 珍珠
5. Zhu Sha (Cinnabaris) 朱砂

Name	Property	CN	Actions & Indications	Remarks
Ci Shi (Magnetitum) 磁石 Magnetite	Salty Acrid Cold	KI LR HT	1. **Calms spirit (Shen):** for insomnia, palpitation, anxiety, and epilepsy due to Kidney Deficiency, Liver Fire disturbing Heart Shen. 2. **Subdues Liver Yang:** for Liver Yang rising manifested as dizziness, irritability, to be angry easily; used with Long Gu, Mu Li. 3. **Improves hearing and**	**15-30g**. Break it to small pieces and decocte 30 minutes longer than other herbs.

			vision: for hearing loss due to Kidney Deficiency and blurred vision due to Kidney and Liver Deficiency. 4. **Calms wheezing:** it can help Kidney to grasp Qi for wheezing due to Kidney Deficiency; used with Dai Zhe Shi, Wu Wei Zi, Hu Tao Ren.	
Long Gu (Os Draconis) 龙骨 Dragon's Bone	Sweet Neutral	HT LR KI	1. **Calms spirit (Shen):** for (1) restlessness, palpitation, forgetfulness, dream disturbed sleep. (2) Epilepsy and convulsion; used with Yuan Zhi, Gui Ban, Suan Zao Ren. 2. **Subdues Liver-Yang:** for Liver Yang rising manifested as dizziness, irritability, easily to be angry; used with Mu Li, Niu Xi, Dai Zhe Shi. 3. **Binds leaking:** for leaking disorders such as spermatorrhea, enuresis, frequent urination, excessive vaginal discharge, spontaneously sweating and night sweating; used with Mu Li, Shan Zhu Yu, Qian Shi.	**15-30g** **Raw Long Gu** calms the spirit. **Calcined Long Gu** is astringent for leakage of fluids and non-healing sores.
Hu Po (Succinum Amber) 琥珀 Amber	Sweet Neutral	BL HT LR	1. **Calms spirit (Shen):** for restlessness, insomnia, palpitation and epilepsy. 2. **Moves Blood and dissipates stasis:** for	**1.5-3g** **Taken as powder without decocting. Do not take it too much.**

			injury, amenorrhea, chest pain and mass. 3. **Promotes urination:** for Lin syndrome and urinary retention.	
Zhen Zhu (Margarita) 珍珠 Pearl	Sweet Salty Cold	HT LR	1. **Calms spirit (Shen):** for (1) restlessness, palpitation, forgetfulness, disturbed sleep with dream. (2) Epilepsy and convulsion. 2. **Improves vision:** for red swollen eyes, blurred vision due to Liver Fire. 3. **Clears Heat and regenerates tissue:** for mouth sore, throat ulcer, and carbuncle.	**0.3-1g**
Zhu Sha (Cinnabaris) 朱砂 Cinnabar	Sweet Cool **Toxic**	HT	1. **Calms spirit (Shen):** for (1) restlessness, insomnia, palpitation due to Heart Fire, Heart Yin and Heart Blood Deficiency; used with Huang Lian, Gan Cao, Dang Gui, Bai Zi Ren, Suan Zao Ren (2) for convulsion and epilepsy due to Wind Heat or Phlegm Heat; used with Hai Ge Ke, Xi Jiao. 2. **Clears Heat toxicity:** Topically use as a powder for carbuncle, sore throat and mouth sore used topically.	**0.1-0.5g per time as powder.** **It is toxic because there is mercury in it!** **Do not decoct it with Fire which makes more mercury coming out.**

Section 2 Herbs that Nourish Heart and Calm Spirit (Shen)

1. Suan Zao Ren (Semen Ziziphi Spinosae) 酸枣仁
2. Bai Zi Ren (Semen Platycladi) 柏子仁
3. Yuan Zhi (Radix Polygalae) 远志
4. He Huan Pi (Cortex Albiziae) 合欢皮
5. Ye Jiao Teng/Shou Wu teng (Caulis Polygoni Multiflori) 夜交藤
6. Ling Zhi (Ganoderma) 灵芝

Name	Property	CN	Actions & Indications	Remarks
Suan Zao Ren (Semen Ziziphi Spinosae) 酸枣仁 Sour Jujube Seed	Sweet Neutral Sour	GB HT LR SP	**1. Calms spirit (Shen):** for insomnia, palpitation, forgetfulness, dream disturbed sleep with dizziness due to Heart and Liver Yin and Blood Deficiency; used with Chuan Xiong, Fu Ling, Zhi Mu (as Suan Zao Ren Tang). **2. Stops sweating:** for spontaneous and night sweating due to Qi or Yin Deficiency; used with Long Gu, Wu Wei Zi, Mu Li.	10-15g as decoction; 1.5-3g as powder.
Bai Zi Ren (Semen Platycladi) 柏子仁 Arbor Vitae Seed, Biota Seed	Sweet Neutral	HT KI LI	**1. Calms spirit (Shen):** for insomnia, palpitation, forgetfulness, dream disturbed sleep with dizziness due to Heart Yin and Blood Deficiency or Heart and Kidney disharmony; used with Yan Zhi, Suan Zao Ren. **2. Moistens Intestine:** for constipation due to large Intestine Dryness; used with Xin Ren, Tao Ren, Chen Pi ,	10-20g Contraindicat-ed in cases with loose stools.

			Song Ren (as Wu Ren Wan). **3. Stops night sweating:** for night sweating due to Heart Yin Deficiency; used with Mu Li, Wu Wei Zi. **4. For hair loss.**	
Yuan Zhi (Radix Polygalae) 远志 Senega root	Bitter Acrid Slighyly Warm	HT LU	**1. Calms spirit (Shen):** for insomnia, palpitation, forgetfulness due to Heart and Kidney disharmony; used with Suan Zao Ren. **2. Resolves Phlegm and opens orifice:** for epilepsy, mania, convulsion due to Phlegm covering clear orifice; used with Yu Jin, Shi Chang Pu. **3. Resolves Phlegm and stops cough:** for cough due to Phlegm; used with Chuan Bei Mu, Ban Xia. **4. Reduces abscess and swelling:** for carbuncle, mastitis, topically use.	5-15g Contraindicat-ed with peptic ulcer and gastritis. According to morden research, it is contraindicat-ed with pregnancy.
He Huan Pi (Cortex Albiziae) 合欢皮 Mimosa Tree Bark	Sweet Neutral	HT LR	**1. Calms spirit (Shen)and soothes Liver Qi:** for insomnia anxiety, restlessness and depression. It is good at calm Shen and relieves depression; used with Dan Shen, Ye Jiao Teng, Bai Zi Ren. **2. Moves Blood and reduces swelling:** for traumatic injury, bone fracture, carbuncle and Lung abscess; used with Ru Xiang, Mo Yao.	10-15g
Ye Jiao Teng/Shou Wu	Sweet Slightly	HT LR	**1. Calms spirit (Shen):** for insomnia due to Heart Yin and	9-15g

Teng (Caulis Polygoni Multiflori) 夜交藤/首乌藤 Polygonum Vine, Fleeceflower Vine Vine of He Shou Wu	Bitter Neutral		Blood Deficiency; used with Suan Zao Ren, Bai Zi Ren. **2. Unblocks channels:** For Bi syndrome due to Wind Dampness with Blood Deficiency; used with Dang Gui, Ji Xue Teng, Dan Shen. **3. Expels Wind and stops itching:** for itching due to Wind Dampness, externally wash.	
Ling Zhi (Ganoderma) 灵芝 Ganoderma, Lucid Ganoderma, Reishi Mushroom	Sweet	HT LR LU	**1. Calms spirit (Shen):** for insomnia due to Heart and Spleen Deficiency, or Qi and Blood Deficiency; used along or with Suan Zao Ren, Long Yan Rou. **2. Stops cough and calms wheezing:** for cough and wheezing due to Phlegm Dampness or Cold Phlegm. **3. Tonifies Qi:** for shortness of breath, fatigue, poor appetite, loose stool due to Spleen Qi Deficiency, or weakness and soreness of lower back and knee, dizziness due to Kidney and Liver Deficiency.	6-12g as decoction; 1.5-3g as powder. The broken spore of Ling Zhi is the best.

Practice 26

1. Long Gu and Mu Li are usually:
A. Decocted 20-30 minutes before adding other substances.
B. Decocted 10 minutes later than other substances.
C. Decocted with other substances.
D. Dissolved in the boiled decoction.

2. Which of the following herbs is the best for palpitations, insomnia, impaired memory, profuse dreams, and abnormal sweating?
A. He Huan Pi
B. Yuan Zhi
C. Ye Jiao Teng
D. Suan Zao Ren

3. Which of the following spirit-calming herbs also invigorates the Blood and stops pain?
A. He Huan Pi
B. Ye Jiao Teng
C. Yuan Zhi
D. Suan Zao Ren

4. Besides nourishing the Heart and calming spirit, Bai Zi Ren also:
A. Clears Liver and strengthens Spleen.
B. Cools the Blood and expels Dampness.
C. Moistens Intestines and relieves constipation.
D. Reduces swelling and dissipates nodules.

5. Which of the following herbs is usually used in powder or pill form?
A. Xiang Fu
B. Huo Xiang
C. Ru Xiang
D. She Xiang

6. Which of the following spirit-calming herbs also binds leaking?
A. Long Gu
B. Dai Zhe Shi
C. Mu Li
D. Yuan Zhi

Answer Keys: 1A. 2D. 3A. 4C. 5D. 6A

Chapter 14 Herbs that Tonify Deficiency

Classification:

1. Herbs that tonify Qi
2. Herbs that tonify Blood
3. Herbs that tonify Yang
4. Herbs that tonify Yin

Section 1 Herbs that Tonify Qi

Common characters:

1. Most of them go to SP channel.
2. Most of them are sweet.
3. May cause fullness in the Middle Jiao if given too much.

Herbs:

1. Ren Shen (Radix Ginseng) 人参
2. Xi Yang Shen (Radix panacis Quinquefolii) 西洋参
3. Dang Shen (Radix Codonopsis Pilosulae) 党参
4. Tai Zi Shen (Radix pseudo-stellariae) 太子参
5. Huang Qi (Radix Astragali seu Hedysari) 黄芪
6. Bai Zhu (Rhizoma Atractylodis Macroceph) 白术
7. Shan Yao (Rhizoma Dioscoreae) 山药
8. Ci Wu Jia (Radix Sev Caulis Acanthopanacis Senticosi) 刺五加
9. Jiao Gu Lan (Rhizoma Beu Herba Gynostemmatis) 绞股蓝
10. Hong Jing Tian (Herba Rhodiolae) 红景天
11. Da Zao (Fructus Ziziphi Jujubae) 大枣
12. Gan Cao (Radix Glycyrrhizae) 甘草
13. Yi Tang (Saccharum Granorum) 饴糖
14. Feng Mi (Mel) 蜂蜜
15. Huang Jing (Polygonati Rhizoma) 黄精

Name	Property	CN	Actions & Indications	Remarks
Ren Shen (Radix Ginseng) 人参 Ginseng root	Sweet Slightly Bitter Slightly Warm	LU SP	1. **Powerfully tonifies Yuan Qi:** for Qi collapse. Now it is used for Heart failure and shock. A. Due to severe or prolonged illness, used alone in large dosage (as Du Shen Tang) B. Due to Deficiency of Qi accompanied with Yang Deficiency, used with Fu Zi (as Shen Fu Tang). 2. **Tonifies Lung:** for Lung Qi Deficiency manifested as shortness of breath and wheezing, whispering voice, weak pulse and spontaneous sweating; used with Huang Qi Wu Wei Zi. 3. **Tonifies Spleen:** for fatigue, poor appetite, loose stool due to Spleen Qi Deficiency; used with Bai Zhu, Fu Ling, Gan Cao (as Si Jun Zi Tang). 4. **Generates fluid and stops thirst:** for thirst due to febrile diseases or diabetes. A. Wasting and thirsting disorder (diabetes), Used with Sheng Di Huang, Mai Men Dong. B. Profuse sweating, thirst, shortness of breath, feeble pulse, Used with Mai Dong, Wu Wei Zi (as Sheng Mai Yin). 5. **Benefits Heart and calms shen:** for insomnia, palpitation and poor memory; used with	5-10g decocted separately or 1.5-2g as powder. 15-30g for shock or Heart failure. **Incompatible with Li Lu and Wu Ling Zi.** Do not take it with Lai Fu Zi, white radish and tea.

			Dang Gui, Zao Ren, Long Yan. Rou (as in Gui Pi Tang).	
Xi Yang Shen (Radix panacis Quinquefolii) 西洋参 American ginseng	Sweet Cold Slightly Bitter	LU ST HT	1. **Benefits Qi and nourishes Yin:** for cough, wheezing with Phlegm and Blood due to Yin Deficiency. 2. **Clears Fire and generates fluid:** for fatigue, thirsty due to Qi and Yin Deficiency from febrile diseases.	**3-6g** decocted separately.It is for Qi and Yin Deficiency. **Incompatible with Li Lu.** Do not use iron pot to decoct it.
Dang Shen (Radix Codonopsis Pilosulae) 党参 Codonopsis root	Sweet Neutral	LU SP	1. **Tonifies Qi and benefits the middle:** for poor appetite, loose stool, fatigue due to Spleen Qi Deficiency. with Bai Zhu, Fu Ling, Gan Cao (as Si Jun Zi Tang). 2. **Tonifies Lung:** for shortness of breath, cough and wheezing, whispered voice due to Lung Qi Deficiency; used with Huang Qi, Wu Wei Zi. 3. **Generates fluid and stops thirst:** for thirst due to febrile diseases or diabetes; used with Wu Wei Zi, Mai Dong. 4. **Tonifies Blood:** for pale face, dizziness and palpitation due to Qi and Blood Deficiency.	**10-30g Incompatible with Li Lu.**
Tai Zi Shen (Radix pseudo-stellariae) 太子参 Pseudostellaria	Sweet Slightly Bitter Neutral	LU SP	1. **Tonifies Qi and benefits Spleen:** for poor appetite, fatigue due to Spleen Deficiency with Stomach Yin Deficiency. 2. **Generates fluid:** for dry cough, palpitation, insomnia and night or spontaneous sweating.	**10-30g Incompatible with Li Lu.**
Huang Qi	Sweet	LU	1. **Tonifies Qi and raises Yang:**	10-15g. Can

(Radix Astragali seu Hedysari) 黄芪 Astragalus root	Slightly Warm	SP	for shortness of breath, poor appetite, loose stool, fatigue due to Spleen Qi Deficiency; or abdominal pain due to Middle Jiao deficient Cold; fatigue with sweating due to Qi and Yang Deficiency; and sinking syndromes such as prolapse of anus and inner organs. A. Spleen Qi Deficiency syndrome, used with Bai Zhu B. Lung Qi Deficiency syndrome. C. General Qi Deficiency after an illness; used with Ren Shen D. Both Qi and Blood Deficiency, with Dang Gui (as Dang Gui Bu Xu Tang). E. Sinking of the middle Qi, used with Ren Shen, Bai Zhu, Sheng Ma , Chai Hu, Dang Gui, Jie Geng (as Bu Zhong Yi Qi Tang). 2. **Tonifies protective (Wei) Qi and stabilizes the Exterior:** for spontaneous sweating, easily to get Cold due to Lung and defensive Qi Deficiency. A. Spontaneous sweating due to Qi Deficiency; used with Bai Zhu, Fang Feng (as Yu Ping Feng San). B. Night sweating due to Yin Deficiency; used with Sheng Di, Huang Bai, Huang Qin, Huang Lian, Dang Gui (as Dang Gui Liu Huang Tang).	be used up to 120g if necessary. **Dry-fried Huang Qi** or honey-fry is good at tonifying Qi and raisng Yang. The **raw Huang Qi** is good for abscesses.

			3. **Promotes urination and reduces edema:** for edema due to Spleen Deficiency with water retention; used with Fang Ji, Bai Zhu (as Fang Ji Huang Qi Tang). 4. **Promotes discharge of pus and generates flesh:** for carbuncles with pus but difficult to open; or can not recover after long time pus discharging. A. Non-formed pus, Used with Chuan Shan Jia, Dang Gui, Zao Jiao Ci (as Tou Nong San). B. No healing, Used with Dang Gui, Ren Shen, Bai Zhu, Shu Di (Shi Quan Da Bu Wan).	
Bai Zhu (Rhizoma Atractylodis Macroceph) 白术 Atractylodes (White) Rhizome	Sweet Bitter Warm	SP ST	1. **Tonifies Qi:** for poor appetite, loose stool, abdominal distention, low energy due to Spleen Qi Deficiency; used with Ren Shen, Fu Ling, Gan Cao (as Si Ju Zi Tang). 2. **Promotes urination:** for edema, urinary retention, Phlegm accumulation due to Spleen Qi Deficiency; used with Fu Ling, Zhu Ling, Ze Xie, Gui Zhi (as Wu Ling San). 3. **Stabilizes the Exterior:** for night or spontaneous sweating due to Spleen Qi Deficiency; used with Huang Qi, Fang Feng (as Yu Ping Feng San). 4. **Calms fetus:** for restless fetus due to Spleen Qi Deficiency. with Dang Shen.	10-15g **Raw Bai Zhu** for Dampness, and **dry-fried Bai Zhu** to strengthen Spleen and tonify Qi.
Shan Yao	Sweet	KI	1. **Tonifies Qi and nourishes Yin:**	10-30g

(Rhizoma Dioscoreae) 山药 Chinese Yam	Neutral	LU SP	for diarrhea, poor appetite due to Spleen Qi Deficiency; used with Ren Shen, Bai Zhu, Fu Ling, Bian Dou (as Shen Ling Bai Zhu San). 2. **Tonifies Lung and Kidney:** for cough, wheezing, spermatorrhea, frequent urination due to Spleen, Lung and Kidney Qi Deficiency; used with Mai Dong, Wu Wei Zi.	Can be used up to 250g if necessary. Use raw herb to tonify the Yin and dry-fried one to strengthen the Spleen.
Ci Wu Jia (Radix Sev Caulis Acantho-panacis Senticosi) 刺五加 Eleuthero root, Siberian ginseng	Pungent Slightly Bitter Warm	SP KI HT	1. **Tonifies Spleen and Lung Qi:** for fatigue, poor appetite, coughing due to Spleen and Lung Qi Deficiency. 2. **Tonifies Kidney and strengthens lower back:** for soreness and pain of lower back, impotence, children retardation of walk, and due to Kidney Deficiency, or Bi syndrome with Liver and Kidney Deficiency. 3. **Tonifies Spleen and Heart, calms Shen:** for insomnia, forgetfulness due to Spleen and Heart Deficiency.	9-20g
Jiao Gu Lan (Rhizoma Beu Herba Gynostemmatis) 绞股蓝 Five-leaf Ginseng, Miracle Grass, Fairy Herb or Southern	Bitter Sweet Cold	SP LU	1. **Tonifies Spleen Qi:** for fatigue, poor appetite due to Spleen Qi Deficiency. Because of its Cold property and it is able to generate fluid and stop thirst, it is good for both Qi and Yin Deficiency such as diabetes manifested as thirst, dry mouth and throat. 2. **Resolves Phlegm and stops**	10-20g decocted. Also can be taken like tea.

Ginseng.			**coughing:** for coughing due to Lung Qi Deficiency with Phlegm obstruct Lung Qi. It can benefit Lung, clear Lung Heat, resolve Phlegm and stop cough. 3. **Resolves toxicity:** for cancer, ulcer.	
Hong Jing Tian (Herba Rhodiolae) 红景天 Roseroot	Sweet Astringent Cold	SP LU	1. **Tonifies Spleen Qi:** for fatigue, due to Spleen Qi Deficiency, leukorrhea due to Spleen Qi Deficiency with Dampness. 2. **Stops cough:** for cough with thick Phlegm or with Blood due to Lung Heat or Lung Yin Deficiency. 3. **Moves Blood:** for Blood stasis, injury, burning.	3-9g
Da Zao (Fructus Ziziphi Jujubae) 大枣 Jujube	Sweet Neutral	SP ST	1. **Tonifies Spleen Qi:** for poor appetite, loose stool, low energy due to Spleen Qi Deficiency. with Dang Shen, Bai Zhu 2. **Nourishes Blood and calms spirit:** for pale face and hysteria (Zhang Zhao) due to Blood Deficiency; used with Gan Cao, Fu Xiao Mai (as Gan Mai Da Zao Tang). 3. **Moderates and harmonizes other herbs:** for reducing side effects and protect upright Qi. Such as Ting Li Da Zao Xie Fei Tang and Shi Zao Tang.	**10-30g** Contraindicat-ed with parasites, food stagnation, and Dampness disorder.
Gan Cao (Radix Glycyrrhizae) 甘草 Licorice root	Sweet Neutral or Sweet Warm	HT LU SP ST	1. **Tonifies Qi and benefits the middle:** for palpitation, intermittent pulse, and fatigue, poor appetite, diarrhea A. Spleen Qi Deficiency, used with Ren Shen, Bai Zhu, Fu	3-10g Use **raw Gan Cao** to clear Heat and relieve toxicity, and

			Ling (as Si Jun Zi Tang). B. Heart Qi Deficiency, with Ren Shen, Gui Zhi, Mai Dong, Sheng Di, Da Zao (as Zhi Gan Cao Tang). **2. Stops cough:** for cough, wheezing whatever Cold or hot, deficient or Excess syndrome; used with Ma Huang, Xing Ren (San Ao Tang or Ma Xing Shi Gan Tang). **3. Moderates spasm and alleviates pain:** for spasmodic pain; used with Shao Yao (as Shao Yao Gan Cao Tang). **4. Clears Heat toxicity:** for carbuncles, sore throat, drug or food poisoning. A. Carbuncles, sores and other skin infections, used with Jin Yin Hua, Lian Qiao. B. Sore throat, used with Jie Geng (as Jie Geng Tang). C. Food and drug poisoning, used with Lu Dou. **5. Moderates and harmonizes other herbs:** for reducing side effects of other herbs and protect SP and ST. A; used in a formula to reduce the toxicity of other herbs or moderate the Cold or hot properties and coordinate the effects of different herbs. B. Guide and conduct other herbs into the channels.	**honey-fry Gan Cao** to tonify the middle and moderate spasms. **Incompatible with Hai Zao, Da Ji, Yuan Hua and Gan Sui.**
Yi Tang	Sweet	LU	**1. Tonifies Spleen Qi:** for poor	**15-30g**

(Saccharum Granorum) 饴糖 Maltose	Slightly Warm	SP ST	appetite, low energy due to Spleen Qi Deficiency. **2. Moderates spasm and alleviates pain:** for deficient Cold abdominal pain. **3. Moistens Lung and stops cough:** for cough due to Lung Dryness.	
Feng Mi (Mel) 蜂蜜 Honey	Sweet Neutral	LU SP LI	**1. Tonifies Qi and relaxes spasm:** for abdominal pain. **2. Moistens Lung and large Intestine:** for dry cough and constipation. **3. Resolves toxicity:** for reducing toxicity of all kinds of Wu Tou.	15-30g
Huang Jing (Polygonati Rhizoma) 黄精 Polygonatum Sibericum, Solomon's Seal root Ophipogon root	Sweet Neutral	KI LU SP	**1. Tonifies Qi and Yin:** for poor appetite, low energy due to Spleen Qi Deficiency. With Ren Shen, Dang Shen, Bai Zhu or Sha Shen, Mai Men Dong. **2. Moistens Lung:** for dry cough due to Kidney Yin Deficiency and Lung Dryness. A. Dry cough with little sputum due to consumption, used with Sha Shen, Zhi Mu. B. Kidney essence Deficiency, used with Xu Duan. **3. Tonified Kidney essence:** for dizziness, lower back and knee soreness, gray hair due to Kidney essence Deficiency; used With Xu Duan.	**10-30g**

Practice 27

1. The patient with pale face due to Blood Deficiency, with dizziness, palpitation, poor appetite and diarrhea should be treated by:
A. Dang Gui
B. Shou Di Huang
C. Dang Shen
D. Bai Shou Yao

2. Which of the following herbs is often used to rescue the collapsed Qi?
A. Dang Shen
B. Yi Mu Cao
C. Ren Shen
D. Huang Qi

3. The herb that tonifies Qi and lifts sinking Yang, strengthens Wei Qi to stops sweating, induces urination to reduce edema is:
A. Huang Qi
B. Dang Shen
C. Gan Cao
D. Da Zao

4. The functions of Bai Zhu are:
A. Tonify SP Qi and lift sinking Yang Qi, nourish Blood and calm spirit.
B. Promote Blood circulation to remove Blood stasis, stop cough and relieve asthma
C. Tonify SP Qi and lift sinking Yang Qi, promote flow of Qi and moisten bowels.
D. Tonify Qi and strengthen SP, induce urination and drain Dampness, stabilize Exterior to stop sweating.

5. Which of the following herbs has the function of promote pus discharge and tissue regeneration?
A. Dang Shen
B. Huang Qi
C. Shan Yao
D. Bai Zhu

6. Which of the following herbs can tonify Qi, and nourish Yin as well?
A. Shan Yao
B. Gan Cao

C. Dang Shen
D. Huang Qi

7. The properties of Ren Shen are:
A. Sweet, bitter, slightly warm.
B. Sweet, slightly warm.
C. Sweet, slightly bitter, warm.
D. Sweet, slightly bitter, slight warm.

8. Bai Zhu treats which kind of sweating:
A. Due to Yang collapse.
B. Due to Qi Deficiency.
C. Due to Yin Deficiency.
D. Due to excessive Heat

9. Which of the following herb can treat SP and LU Qi Deficiency, with shallow respiration, shortness of breath, sweating and lassitude of extremities is?
A. Huang Qi
B. Dang Shen
C. Ren Shen
D. He Shou Wu

10. Gan Cao enters:
A. HT LU SP and ST channels
B. HT and ST channels
C. LU, SP and LV channels
D. SP and HT channels

11. Which of the following herbs is sweet, warm, and has the functions of tonifying Qi and strengthening the Middle Jiao, nourishing Blood and calming spirit, relieving toxins of other herbs?
A. Huang Qi
B. Da Zao
C. Dang Shen
D. Gan Cao

12. Which of following herbs treat cough, and muscle spasm?
A. Shan Yao
B. Dang Shen
C. Bai Shao Yao

D. Gan Cao

13. Which of the following Qi tonics can also clear Heat and Fire toxins to treat carbuncles and sores?
A. Huang Qi
B. Bai Zhu
C. Gan Cao
D. Ren Shen

Answer Keys: 1C. 2C. 3A. 4D. 5B. 6A. 7D. 8B. 9A. 10A. 11B. 12D. 13C

Section 2 Herbs that Tonify Yang

Common characters:

5. All of them are warm or hot.
6. All of them go to KI channel.
7. Contraindicated in Yin Deficiency Fire.

Herbs:

1. Lu Rong (Cornu Cervi Pantotrichum) 鹿茸
2. Lu Jiao Jiao (Cervi Cornus Colla) 鹿角胶
3. Ba Ji Tian (Radix Morindae Officinalis) 巴戟天
4. Yin Yang Huo (Herba Epimedii) 淫羊藿
5. Xian Mao (Rhizoma Curculiginis) 仙茅
6. Bu Gu Zhi (Fructus Psoraleae) 补骨脂
7. Yi Zhi Ren (Fructus Alpiniae Oxyphyllae) 益智仁
8. Tu Si Zi (Semen Cuscutae) 菟丝子
9. Sha Yuan Ji Li (Semen Astragali Complanati) 沙苑蒺藜
10. Rou Cong Rong (Herba Cistanchis) 肉苁蓉
11. Suo Yang (Herba Cynomorri Songgarici) 锁阳
12. Du Zhong (Cortex Eucommiae) 杜仲
13. Xu Duan (Radix Dipsaci Asperi) 续断
14. Ge Jie (Gecko) 蛤蚧
15. Dong Chong Xia Cao (Cordyceps) 冬虫夏草
16. Zi He Che (Placenta Hominis) 紫河车
17. Hu Lu Ba (Semen Trigonellae) 胡芦巴
18. Hu Tao Ren / He Tao Ren (Semen Juglandis) 胡/核桃仁
19. Gu Sui Bu (Rhizoma Drynariae) 骨碎补
20. Jiu Cai Zi (Semen Allii Tuberosi) 韭菜子
21. Hai Gou Shen (Testes et Penis Callorhini Seu Phocae) 海狗肾
22. Yang Qi Shi (Actinolitum) 阳起石
23. Hai Ma (Hippocampus) 海马
24. Xiong Can E (Bombyx Masculus) 雄蚕娥

Name	Property	CN	Actions & Indications	Remarks
Lu Rong (Cornu Cervi Pantotrichum)	Sweet Salty Warm	KI LR	1. **Tonifies Kidney Yang:** For impotence, frequent urination, infertility, dizziness, tinnitus, lower	**1-3g**. Take as powder. Start from 1g

鹿茸 Elk/Deer Horn, Velvet Young antler of deer			back and knee pain; used alone or with Ren Shen, Shan Yao, Bu Gu Zhi. 2. **Augments essence, and strengthens sinew and bone:** for child physiological and mental development retardation; used with Shu Di, Shan Yao, Shan Zhu Yu. 3. **Regulates Chong and Ren, and stabilize Girdle:** for uterine bleeding and excessive vaginal discharge due to Deficiency Cold of Chong and Ren channels. 4. **Resolves toxicity:** for Yin type boils, used with Huang Qi.	and gradually increase. Contraindicated in syndrome with Heat from Yin Deficiency, Heat in the Blood level. Contraindicated in case of Phlegm-Heat, or Fire or warm-febrile diseases.
Lu Jiao Jiao (Cervi Cornus Colla) 鹿角胶 Deer Antler Glue	Sweet Salty	KI LR	1. **Tonifies Liver and Kidney** 2. **Nourishes Blood and essence** 3. **Stops bleeding**	Deer antler glue 5-10g
The following 3 herbs can **tonify Kidney Yang and Strengthen bone and sinew; expel Wind-Damp-Cold for Bi syndrome.**				
Ba Ji Tian (Radix Morindae Officinalis) 巴戟天 Morinda root	Acrid Sweet Warm	KI LR	1. **Tonifies Kidney Yang:** for impotence, irregular menstruation, infertility, lower abdominal Cold and pain; used with Suo Yang, Yin Yang Huo, Rou Cong Rong. 2. **Strengthens bone and sinew, expel Wind-Damp-Cold:** for Bi syndrome; used with Du Zhong, Xu Duan, Niu Xi.	10-15g It is less hot than Yin Yang Huo and Xian Mao. It can also consume Kidney essence.
Yin Yang Huo (Herba Epimedii) 淫羊藿 (Xian Ling	Acrid Sweet Warm	KI LR	1. **Tonifies Kidney Yang:** for impotence, spermatorrhea, infertility, frequent urination; used with Xian Mao, Ba Ji Tian. 2. **Strengthens bone and sinew, expels Wind-Damp-Cold:** for Bi	5-10g It is stronger to tonify Yang than Ba Ji Tian and Xian Mao. It can increase sperm.

Pi) （仙灵脾，三枝九叶草，弃杖草） Arial Parts of Epimedium			syndrome; used with Chuan Xiong, Du Zhong. **3. Stops cough and calms wheezing:** for cough and wheezing.	It can consume Kidney essence.
Xian Mao (Rhizoma Curculiginis) 仙茅 Golden Eye Grass Rhizome	Acrid Hot **Toxic**	KI LR	**1. Tonifies Kidney Yang, controls essence and urine:** for impotence, urinary incontinence, frequent urination; used with Du Zhong, Yin Yang Huo. **2. Strengthens bone and sinew, expels Wind-Damp-Cold:** for Bi syndrome; used with Du Zhong, Du Huo. **3. Warms Spleen Yang and stops diarrhea:** for diarrhea, Cold abdominal pain; used with Gan Jiang, Bai Zhu. 4. Regulates menstruation and menopause.	3-10g It can consume Kidney essence. 1. Contraindicated in cases of Yin Deficiency with Heat signs 2. Long term use is not recommended 3. Toxic reactions include swelling of the tongue.
The following 4 herbs can **tonify Kidney Yang and keep Kidney Qi**. All of them are seeds.				
Bu Gu Zhi (Fructus Psoraleae) 补骨脂（破故纸） Psoralea Fruit	Acrid Bitter Very Warm	KI SP	**1. Tonifies Kidney Yang:** for impotence, soreness and weak knee and lower back. with Du Zhong, Hu Tao Ren. **2. Stabilizes essence and urine:** for spermatorrhea, frequent urination; used with Sang Piao Xiao, Yi Zhi Ren, Fu Pen Zhi. **3. Warms Spleen:** for diarrhea due to Spleen and Kidney Yang Deficiency. with Rou Dou Kou, Wu Wei Zi, Wu Zhu Yu (as Si Shen Wan). **4. Helps Kidney to grasp Qi:** for chronic coughing and wheezing due	6-15g Contraindicated in deficient Yin with Heat signs or constipation.

			to Kidney and Lung Deficiency. with Ren Shen, Hu Tao Ren, Wu Wei Zi.	
Yi Zhi Ren (Fructus Alpiniae Oxyphyllae) 益智仁 Black Cardamon Fruit	Acrid Warm	KI SP	1. **Tonifies Kidney Yang, controls essence and urine:** for impotence, frequent urination, poor memory. with Wu Yao, Shan Yao. 2. **Warms Spleen Yang and controls salivation:** for diarrhea, Cold abdominal pain and excessive salivation; used with Dang Shen, Ban Xia, Fu ling, Bai Zhu and Gan Jiang.	3-10g Contraindicated in case of Heat syndrome.
Tu Si Zi (Semen Cuscutae) 菟丝子 Chinese Dodder Seeds	Acrid Sweet Neutral	KI LR	1. **Tonifies Kidney Yang, controls essence and urine:** for impotence, spermatorrhea, urinary incontinence, frequent urination, excessive vaginal discharge. A. Lower back pain, tinnitus, impotence, used with Du Zhong, Gou Qi Zi. B. Nocturnal emission, frequent urination, leukorrhea, used with Fu Peng Zi, Wu Wei Zi. 2. **Tonifies Liver and improves vision:** for blurred vision, due to Kidney and Liver Deficiency; used with Gou Qi Zi, Ju Hua, Sha Yuan, Ji Li. 3. **Warms Spleen Yang and stops diarrhea:** for diarrhea, Cold abdominal pain due to Spleen and Kidney Deficiency; used with Lian Zi Rou, Shan Yao, Fu Ling (as Tu Si Zi Wan). 4. **Calms fetus:** for restless fetus, bleeding during pregnancy; used	10-15g Caution in cases of Yin Deficiency with Heat signs. It has estrogen like action.

			with Xu Duan, Sang Ji Sheng, E Jiao (as in Shou Tai Wan). 5. **For diabetes due to Kidney Deficiency.**	
Sha Yuan Ji Li (Semen Astragali Complanati) 沙苑蒺藜 Milkvetch Seed, Astragalus Seed	Sweet Warm	KI LR	1. **Tonifies Kidney Yang, controls essence and urine:** for impotence, spermatorrhea, premature ejaculation, urinary incontinence, frequent urination, excessive vaginal discharge, lower back pain; used with Fu Pen Zi, Qian Shi, Lian Zi. 2. **Tonifies Liver and improves vision:** for blurred vision; used with Gou Qi Zi, Shu Di Huang.	10-15g
The following 2 herbs can **tonify Kidney Yang and Moisten Intestine**.				
Rou Cong Rong (Herba Cistanchis) 肉苁蓉 Fleshy Stem of Broomrape	Sweet Salty Warm	LI KI	1. **Tonifies Kidney Yang:** for impotence, spermatorrhea, infertility, soreness and weak knee and lower back; used with Shu Di, Tu Si Zi, Ba Ji Tian, Du Zhong. 2. **Moistens Intestine:** for constipation due to Yin, Yang or Blood Deficiency; used with Chen Xiang, Huo Ma Ren (as Run Chang Wan).	10-15g up to 60g individually. Contraindicated in diarrhea due to SP Deficiency.
Suo Yang (Herba Cynomorri Songgarici) 锁阳 Fleshy Stem of Cynomorium	Sweet Warm	LI KI LR	1. **Tonifies Kidney Yang:** for impotence, spermatorrhea, infertility, soreness and weak knee and lower back; used with Niu Xi, Tu Si Zi , Du Zhong. 2. **Moistens Intestine:** for constipation due to Yin, Yang or Blood Deficiency; used with Rou Cong Rong.	10-15g Contraindicated in diarrhea due to SP Deficiency.

The following 2 herbs can **tonify Kidney Yang, strengthen bone and sinew and calm fetus**.				
Du Zhong (Cortex Eucommiae) 杜仲 Eucommia Bark	Sweet Slightly Acrid Warm	KI LR	1. **Tonifies Kidney Yang, strengthens bone and sinew:** for impotence, soreness and weak knee and lower back, frequent urination; used with Tu Si Zi, Du Huo. 2. **Calms fetus:** for restless fetus, bleeding during pregnancy; used with Xu Duan, Shan Yao.	10-15g Lowing BP Contraindicated in Heat from Yin Deficiency
Xu Duan (Radix Dipsaci Asperi) 续断 Himalayan Teasel root	Bitter Acrid Slightly Warm	KI LR	1. **Tonified Kidney Yang, strengthens sinews and bones:** for weakness of knee and lower back. Bi syndrome, traumatic injury, bone fracture. 2. **Calms fetus:** for restless fetus, bleeding during pregnancy.	10-15g
The following 3 herbs are not plant origin. They can **tonify Kidney Yang and Lung Qi**. They also can tonify essence and Blood.				
Ge Jie (Gecko) 蛤蚧 Gecko	Salty Neutral	LU KI	1. **Tonifies Kidney Yang:** for impotence due to Kidney Yang and essence Deficiency; used with Ren Shen, Hu Tao Ren, Lu Rong. 2. **Tonifies Kidney and Lung:** for chronic cough and wheezing due to Kidney and Lung Deficiency; used with Hu Tao Ren, Wu Wei Zi, Ren Shen.	3-10g of decoction. 1-2g as powder. Good at cough and wheezing due to KI def.
Dong Chong Xia Cao (Cordyceps) 冬虫夏草 Cordyceps sinensis Berk,Chinese Caterpillar Fungas	Sweet Warm	LU KI	1. **Tonifies Kidney Yang:** for impotence, spermatorrhea; used with Du Zhong, Yin Yang Huo, Rou Cong Rong. 2. **Tonifies Kidney and Lung, stops bleeding:** for chronic cough and wheezing, cough with Blood due to Kidney and Lung Deficiency. A. Due to both Kidney and Lung Deficiency, used with Huang Qi, Hu	5-10g Tonify KI & LU. Used with caution in Exterior conditions.

			Tao Rou. B. Due to Qi and Yin Deficiency, used with E Jiao, Mai Dong, Chuan Bei Mu.	
Zi He Che (Placenta Hominis) 紫河车 Placenta	Sweet Salty Warm	LR KI LU	1. **Tonifies Kidney Yang, controls essence and urine:** for infertility, impotence, spermatorrhea, premature ejaculation, urinary incontinence, dizziness and tinnitus. use alone or with Shu Di, Lu Rong, Dong Chong Xia Cao. **2.** **Tonifies Lung Qi:** for cough and wheezing; used with Wu Wei Zi, Mai Man Dong. **3.** **Tonifies Qi and Blood:** for pale complexion, fatigue, post partum lactation Deficiency. use alone or with Huang Qi, Dang Gui, Bai Zhu, Shan Yao.	**1.5-3g as powder.**
The following herbs are less important as herbs above.				
Hu Lu Ba (Semen Trigonellae) 胡芦巴 Fenugreek seed	Bitter Warm	KI LR	**1.** **Tonifies Kidney Yang:** for impotence, spermatorrhea. **2.** **Disperses Cold Dampness and stops pain:** for hernia pain, lower abdominal pain, and dysmenorrhea.	5-10g
Hu Tao Ren / He Tao Ren (Semen Juglandis) 胡桃仁/核桃仁 Walnut Nut	Sweet Warm	KI LI LU	**1.** **Tonifies Kidney Yang:** for impotence, soreness and weak knee and lower back, frequent urination, hair loss, poor memory. with Du Zhong, Bu Gu Zhi. **2.** **Tonifies Kidney and Lung, helps Kidney to grasp Qi:** for chronic cough and wheezing due to Kidney and Lung Deficiency; used with Ge Jie, Ren Shen. **3.** **Moistens Intestine:** for constipation due to Yin or Blood	**10-30g** Used with caution in cases of loose stool.

			Deficiency; used with Huo Ma Ren, Rou Cong Rong.	
Jiu Cai Zi (Semen Allii Tuberosi) 韭菜子 Chiese Leek Seed	Acrid Sweet Warm	KI LR	1. **Tonifies Kidney Yang, controls essence and urine:** for impotence, spermatorrhea, premature ejaculation, urinary incontinence, frequent urination, excessive vaginal discharge. 2. **Tonifies Kidney and Liver, strengthens sinews and bones:** for weakness of knee and lower back.	5-10g Testosterone like action.
Hai Gou Shen (Testes et Penis Callorhini Seu Phocae) 海狗肾 Male Seal Sexual Organs	Salty Hot	KI LR	1. **Tonifies Kidney Yang, controls essence and urine:** for impotence, spermatorrhea, premature ejaculation, infertility. Use alone or with Dong Chong Xia Cao, Ba Ji Tian.	**1-3g** as powder or put in wine to drink. It has testosterone like action.
Yang Qi Shi (Actinolitum) 阳起石 Actinolite	Salty Slightly Warm	KI	1. **Tonifies Kidney Yang, controls essence and urine:** for impotence, spermatorrhea, premature ejaculation, infertility.	**3-6g** as powder. Contraindicated for pregnancy. It can lead to miscarriage. Testosterone like action.
Hai Ma (Hippocampus) 海马 Sea Horse	Sweet Salty Warm	KI LR	1. **Tonifies Kidney Yang, controls essence and urine:** for impotence, spermatorrhea, premature ejaculation, urinary incontinence, frequent urination; used with Gou Qi Zi, Da Zao. 2. **Moves Blood and resolve mass:** for masses with Yang Deficiency; used with invigorating Blood herbs 3. **Reduces swollen and stops pain:** for	**1-1.5g** It has testosterone like action. Contraindicated for pregnancy because it can lead to miscarriage.

			injury.	
Xiong Can E (Bombyx Masculus) 雄蚕娥	Salty Warm	HT KI	1. **Tonifies Kidney Yang, controls essence and urine:** for infertility, impotence, spermatorrhea, premature ejaculation. 2. **Stops bleeding and generates flesh:** for carbuncles.	6-15g
Hai shen (Stichopus Japonicus) 海参 Sea Cucumber, Sea Slug, Trepang	Salty Warm	HT KI	**1. Tonifies Kidney Yang** **2. Stabilizes essence**	
Hai Long (Hailong) 海龙 Pipe Fish	Sweet Salty Slightly Warm	KI	**1. Tonifies Kidney Yang**	
E guan shi (Stalactitum)	Sweet Warm	LU	**1. Tonifies Yang, direct Qi downward**	

Practice 28

1. Lu Rong is:
A. Pungent, warm.
B. Bitter, warm.
C. Sweet, slight warm.
D. Sweet, salty, warm.

2. The herb with pungent, hot and toxic properties is:
A. Xian Mao
B. Ba Ji Tian
C. Yin Yang Huo
D. Bu Gu Zhi

3. The functions of Yin Yang Huo are:
A. Tonify KI Yang, Strengthen bone and sinew and expel Wind-Damp-Cold.
B. Tonify KI and LV, and warm LU.
C. Tonify Yang, transform Cold Phlegm and dry Dampness.
D. Tonify KI and SP, nourish Blood and moisten LU.

4. The herb that treats impotence due to KI Yang Deficiency, and chronic cough with Bloody Phlegm is:
A. Du Zhong
B. Xing Ren
C. Dong Chong Xia Cao
D. Ba Ji Tian

5. The functions of Du Zhong are:
A. Tonify KI and LV, moisten bowel and stop cough.
B. Tonify KI and LV, strengthen the sinews and bones, and calm the fetus.
C. Tonify KI Yang and expel Wind-Damp.
D. Tonify KI and LU, and calm the fetus.

6. The functions of Lu Rong are:
A. Nourish Blood and body essence, and expel Phlegm.
B. Tonify KI Yang, nourish essence, and strengthen the sinews and bones.
C. Tonify LV and KI, moisten bowel and benefit throat.
D. Tonify KI Yang and induce urination.

7. Which pair of Yang tonifying herb is best to treat low back and knee soreness and weakness due to KI Yang Deficiency?
A. Du Zhong & Tu Si Zi.
B. Du Zhong & Xu Duan.
C. Bu Gu Zi & Xian Mao.
D. Yin Yang Huo & Xian Mao.

8. Which of the following herbs tonifies LV and KI, promotes mending of the sinews and bones, also stops uterine bleeding and calms the fetus?
A. Shu Di Huang.
B. Sha Shen.
C. Xu Duan.
D. Nu Zhen Zi.

9. The herb that tonifies KI and strengthens Yang, and moistens bowel to relieve constipation is:
A. Rou Cong Rong
B. Shu Di Huang
C. He Shou Wu
D. Dang Gu

Answer Keys: 1D. 2A. 3A. 4C. 5B. 6B. 7B. 8C. 9A

Section 3 Herbs that Tonify Blood

Common characters:

They are sweet and may damage Spleen. So they are contraindicated for diarrhea caused by Spleen Deficiency.

Herbs:

1. Dang Gui (Radix Angelicae Sinensis) 当归
2. Shu Di Huang (Radix Rehmanniae Praeparata) 熟地黄
3. Bai Shao(Radix Paeoniae Alba) 白芍
4. He Shou Wu (Radix Polygoni Multiflori) 何首乌
5. E Jiao(Gelatinum Corri Asini) 阿胶
6. Long Yan Rou(Arillus Longan) 龙眼肉

Name	Property	CN	Actions & Indications	Remarks
Dang Gui (Radix Angelicae Sinensis) 当归 Chinese Angelica	Bitter Sweet Acrid Warm	HT SP LR	**1. Nourishes Blood:** for Blood Deficiency. It is one of the important herbs to tonify Blood; used with Bai Shao, Chuan Xiong (as Si Wu Tang and Dang Gui Bu Xue Tang). **2. Moves Blood and regulates menstruation:** for dysmenorrhea, irregular menstruation and amenorrhea with both Blood Deficiency and Blood stasis. A. Due to Blood Deficiency, used with Shu Di, Bai Shao, E Jiao. B. Due to Blood stasis, used with Chuan Xiong, Chi Shao, Tao Ren (as Tao Hong Si Wu Tang). **3. Moves Blood and stops pain:**	5-15g Known as "Women's Ren Shen". It is also moving. Vinegar-frying or wine-frying strengthen its Blood-moving properties.

			for pain due to Blood Deficiency, Blood stasis, Cold, injury, and Wind Cold Dampness. A. Abdominal pain, used with Bai Shao, Gan Cao. B. Traumatic injury pain, used with Da Huang, Tao Ren, Hong Hua (as Fu Yuan Huo Xue Tang). C. Bi syndrome (painful obstruction) due to Wind Damp, used with Gui Zhi, Du Huo, Ji Sheng, Qin Jiao (as Du Huo Ji Sheng Tang). 4. **Nourishes Blood and regenerates flesh:** for carbuncles and boils. A. Early stage, used with Ji Yin Hua, Chi Shao, Bai Zhi, Bei Mu (as Xian Fang Huo Ming Yin). B. Middle sage, used with Chuan Shan Jia, Zao Jiao Ci, Huang Qi (as Tou Nong San). C. Slow-healing after rupture due to Qi and Blood. Deficiency, used with Huang Qi, Shu Di, Bai Shao, Ren Shen, Bai Zhu (as Shi Quan Da Bu Tang). 5. **Moistens Intestine:** for constipation due to Blood Deficiency leading to large Intestine Dryness; used with Rou Cong Rong, Shou Wu, Huo Ma Ren.	
Shu Di Huang	Sweet	HT	1. **Nourishes Blood:** for	**10-30g** up to

(Radix Rehmanniae Praeparata) 熟地黄 Rehmannia, Chinese Foxglove root	Slightly Warm	KI LR	dizziness, palpitation, insomnia, menstruation disorders due to Blood Deficiency. It is one of the important herbs to tonify Blood; used with Bai Shao, Dang Gui, Chuan Xiong (as Si Wu Tang). **2. Nourishes Yin:** for hot flash, steaming bone symptom, lower back soreness, tinnitus, hearing loss, spermatorrhea, Xiao Ke (diabetes) due to Kidney Yin or essence Deficiency; used with Shan Yao, Wu Zhu Yu, Ze Xie (as Liu Wei Di Huang Wan). **3. Nourishes essence:** for lower back and knee soreness, dizziness, tinnitus, gray hair; used with Gui Ban, Bie Jia.	60g 1. Caution in cases of Spleen and Stomach Deficiency and stagnant Qi or Phlegm. 2. Overuse can lead to abdominal distention and loose stools.
Bai Shao (Radix Paeoniae Alba) 白芍 White Peony root	Bitter Sour Cool	LR SP	**1. Nourishes Blood and regulates menses:** for menstruation disorders; used with Di Huang, Chuan Xiong, Dang Gui (as Si Wu Tang). **2. Subdues Liver Yang:** for headache, dizziness; used with Tian Men Tong, Xuan Shen. **3. Stops pain:** hypochondriac pain, abdominal pain with spasm. A. Chest or hypochondriac pain, used with Chai Hu, Xiang Fu (as Chai Hu Shu Gan San). B. Abdominal pain and	10-15g up to 30g It is weak to nourish Blood. It is commonly used to subdue Liver Yang. Dry-fry to nourish the Blood and harmonize the Ying and Wei. Used with caution in cases of diarrhea due

			diarrhea, used with Bai Zhu, Chen Pi, Fang Feng (as Tong Xie Yao Fang). C. Spasm of the abdomen or extremities, used with Gan Cao (as Shao Yao Gan Cao Tang). 4. **Preserves Yin and stops sweating:** for spontaneous and night sweating. A. Due to Yin Deficiency, used with Long Gu, Mu Li. B. Disharmony of Nutritive and protective levels, used with Gui Zhi, Sheng Jiang, Da Zao.	to deficient Cold. Incompatible with **Li Lu.**
He Shou Wu (Radix Polygoni Multiflori) 何首乌 Polygonum root, Fo-Ti, Fleece Flower root	Bitter Sweet Slightly Warm astringent	KI LR	1. **Nourishes Blood and essence:** for dizziness, palpitation, insomnia, fatigue, tinnitus, lower back and knee soreness; used with Gang Gui, Gou Qi Zi, Bai Shao, Nu Zhen Zi, Han Lian Cao. 2. **Blackens hairs:** for gray hair. 3. **Resolves toxicity:** for carbuncles, boils. A. Sores, carbuncles, with Ku Shen, Pu Gong Ying. B. Scrofula, with Xia Ku Cao, Bei Mu, Xuan Shen. C. Goiter, neck lumps, with Hai Zao, Kun Bu. 4. **Moistens Intestine:** for constipation. with Dang Gui, Huo Ma Ren. 5. **Treats malaria:** for malaria. with Ren Shen, Dang Gui, Chen Pi (as He Ren Yin).	**10-30g** Raw He Shou Wu for resolving toxicity, moistening the Intestines and treating malaria. prepared He Shou Wu for tonifying.

E Jiao (Gelatinum Corri Asini) 阿胶 Donkey-Hide Glue, Gelatin	Sweet Neutral	KI LR LU	1. **Nourishes Blood:** for pale complexion, dizziness, palpitation. with Dang Shen, Dang Gui, Shu Di, Huang Qi. 2. **Stops bleeding:** for bleeding especially with Blood and Yin Deficiency. use alone or with Sheng Di, Bai Shao, Ai Ye (as Jiao Ai Tang). 3. **Nourishes Yin and moistens Dryness:** for dry cough, spasmodic contraction of voluntary muscles due to Heat injured Yin; used with Xing Ren, Niu Bang Zi, Ma Dou Ling (as Bu Fei E Jiao Tang).	5-15g Dissolved in hot decoction (Yang Hua 烊化). 1.Contraindicated in cases with Exterior disorders 2. Caution in cases of Spleen and Stomach Deficiency
Long Yan Rou (Arillus Longan) 龙眼肉 Longan Fruit Flesh	Sweet Warm	HT SP	1. **Nourishes Blood and calms spirit (Shen):** for palpitation, insomnia, poor memory due to Heart and Spleen Blood Deficiency; used with Ren Shen, Bai Zhu, Huang Qi, Dang Gui.	10-15g Contraindicated in cases of Phlegm-Fire or Dampness in the Middle-Jiao.

Practice 29

1. The herb that tonifies Blood and promotes Blood circulation, relieves pain, and moistens the bowels as well is:
A. E Jiao
B. Shu Di Huang
C. He Shou Wu
D. Dang Gui

2. The menstruation pain due to Blood Deficiency or Blood stagnation should be treated by:
A. Shu Di Huang
B. Bai Shao Yao
C. Dang Gui
D. Huang Qi

3. Which of the following Blood tonitying herbs also has the function of astringing Yin to stop sweating?
A. Da Zao
B. Bai Shao Yao
C. Long Yan Rou
D. E Jiao

4. The herb that tonifies HT and SP, and calms spirit is:
A. Long Yan Rou
B. Sang Shen
C. Dang Gui
D. Shu Di Huang

5. Which of following functions is NOT He Shou Wu's?
A. Tonify Blood and body essence.
B. Improve Qi circulation
C. Moisten bowel.
D. Tonify essence

6. The herb that tonifies Blood and nourishes Yin, and stops bleeding as well is:
A. Bai Shou yao
B. Chuan Xiong
C. E Jiao
D. Sang Shen

7. White Shao Yao treats diarrhea due to:

A. Spleen Deficiency
B. Food stagnation
C. Kidney Yang Deficiency
D. Damp-Heat retention.

Answer Keys: 1D. 2C. 3B. 4A. 5B. 6C. 7A

Section 4 Herbs that Tonify Yin

Common characters:

1. They are **tonifying** herbs.
2. Most of them are **Cold**, sweet and **bitter**.
3. They can moisten Dryness and clear Heat of certain organ.
4. Inappropriate for SP or ST Deficiency, Dampness, Phlegm or diarrhea.

Herbs:

1. Nan Sha Shen (Radix Adenophorae) 南沙参
2. Bei Sha Shen (Radix Glehniae Littoralis) 北沙参
3. Yu Zhu (Rhizoma Polygonati Odorati) 玉竹
4. Tian (Men) Dong (Radix Asparagi) 天(门)冬
5. Mai (Men) Dong (Radix Ophiopogonis) 麦(门)冬
6. Shi Hu (Herba Dendrobii) 石斛
7. Bai He (Bulbus Lilii) 百合
8. Han Lian Cao/ Mo Han Lian (Herba Ecliptae Prostratae) 墨旱莲
9. Nu Zhen Zi(Fructus Ligustri Lucidi) 女贞子
10. Hei Zhi Ma (Semen Sesami Idici) 黑芝麻
11. Gui Ban (Plasttrum Testudinis) 龟板
12. Bie Jia (Carapax Amydea Sinensis) 鳖甲
13. Gou Qi Zi (Fructus Lycii) 枸杞子
14. Sang Shen (Fructus Mori Albea) 桑椹
15. Yin Er (Fructicato Tremellae) 银耳

Name	Property	CN	Actions & Indications	Remarks
Nan Sha Shen (Radix Adenophorae) Straight Ladybell root 南沙参 Adenophora	Sweet Cool Slightly Bitter	LU ST	1. **Nourishes Lung Yin, clears Lung and expels Phlegm:** for dry cough without or with limited Phlegm, or with sticky Phlegm due to Lung Yin Deficiency or Lung Dryness; used with Mai Dong, Yu Zhu, Sang Ye (as in Sha Shen Mai Dong Tang).	10-15g Good at stopping cough. Incompatible with **Li Lu.** Some doctors believe that it is compatible with Li Lu which was found later than the 18 incompatibilities

			2. **Nourishes Stomach Yin and tonifies Qi:** for dry throat and mouth, constipation, vomiting with red tongue, poor appetite due to Qi and body fluid Deficiency after febrile diseases, or due to Spleen and Stomach Deficiency; used with Sheng Di, Mai Dong, Yu Zhu (as Yi Wei Tang).	were declared. It can also tonify Qi which Bei Sha Shen can not.
Bei Sha Shen 北沙参 (Radix Glehniae Littoralis) Coastal Glehnia root	Sweet Cool Slightly Bitter	LU ST	1. **Nourishes Lung Yin and clears Lung:** for dry cough without or with limited Phlegm, or with sticky Phlegm, dry throat and mouth, loss of voice, hemoptysis due to Lung Yin Deficiency; used with Mai Dong, Yu Zhu, Sang Ye (as Sha Shen Mai Dong Tang). 2. **Nourishes Stomach Yin and generates fluid:** for dry throat and mouth with red tongue, mild Stomach ache, dry vomiting due to Stomach Yin Deficiency or febrile diseases damaged Yin; used with Sheng Di, Mai Dong, Yu Zhu (as Yi Wei Tang).	10-15g It is stronger to Nourish Yin than Nan Sha Shen. **Incompatible with Li Lu.** It is stronger to Nourish Yin than Nan Sha Shen.
Yu Zhu (Rhizoma Polygonati Odorati) 玉竹	Sweet Slightly Cold	LU ST	1. **Nourishes Lung Yin :** for dry cough without or with limited Phlegm, coughing with Blood, dry throat and mouth, loss of voice; used	10-15g; Also called Wei Rui

Solomon's Seal			with Sha Shen, Mai Dong. 2. **Nourishes Stomach Yin and stops thirst:** for dry throat and mouth, poor appetite after febrile diseases that injured body fluid or diabetes.	
Mai (Men) Dong (Radix Ophiopogonis) Ophipogon Ro 麦(门)冬 Dwarf Lilyturf Tuber	Sweet Cool Slightly Bitter	LU ST HT	1. **Nourishes Lung Yin and moistens Lung:** for dry cough with sticky Phlegm, dry nose, sore throat, loss of voice, hemoptysis due to Lung Yin Deficiency; used with Sha Shen, Mai Dong. 2. **Nourishes Stomach Yin and generates fluid:** for thirsty, dry mouth, epigestric pain, poor appetite and constipation due to Stomach Yin Deficiency or Stomach Yin injured by Heat; used with Mai Men Dong, Sha Shen, Sheng Di. 3. **Nourishes Heart Yin and eliminates irritability:** for Heart Yin Deficiency or Ying stage febrile diseases manifested as irritability, memory loss, palpitation, insomnia; used with Bai Wei, Dan Dou Chi, Cong Bai, Jie Geng (as in Tian Wang Bu Xi Dan).	10-15g
Tian (Men) Dong (Radix Asparagi) 天(门)冬	Sweet Bitter Cold	LU KI	1. **Nourishes Lung Yin and clears Lung:** for dry cough or cough with Blood due to Lung Yin Deficiency. A. Dry cough due to	10-15g

Cochinchinese Asparagus root			Dryness of Lung, used with Mai Dong. B. Cough with hemoptysis due to Lung Yin Deficiency and Lung Heat, used with Sheng Di Huang, Mai Dong. 2. **Nourishes Kidney Yin, clears empty Fire and generates fluid:** for hot flash, night sweating, spermatorrhea, diabetes, constipation due to Kidney and body fluid Deficiency; used with Ren Shen, Shu Di Huang, Huang Qi.	
Shi Hu (Herba Dendrobii) 石斛 Dendrobium Stem	Sweet Cold Slightly Salty Bland	ST KI	1. **Nourishes Yin and clears Deficiency Heat:** for low fever, irritability, and thirst due to febrile diseases which injured body fluid; used with Bai Wei. 2. **Nourishes Stomach and generates fluid:** for Stomach Yin Deficiency; used with Sha Shen, Mai Dong, Yu Zhu. 3. **Brightens eyes:** for blurry vision, night blindness due to Kidney and Liver Deficiency; used with Shu Di, Niu Xi, Gou Qi Zi, Gui Ban.	10-15g
Bai He (Bulbus Lilii) 百合 Lily Bulb	Sweet Slightly Cold Slightly Bitter	LU HT	1. **Nourishes Yin and moistens Lung and stops cough:** for dry and chronic cough, cough with Blood. with Kuan Dong Hua, used	**10-30g**

			with Sheng Di, Xuan Shen, Bei Mu (as Bai He Gu Jin Tang). 2. **Clears Heart and calms spirit:** for later stage febrile diseases with low fever, irritability, insomnia; used with Zhi Mu or Sheng Di (as Bei He Zhi Mu Tang or Bai He Di Huang Tang.	
Han Lian Cao/ Mo Han Lian 墨旱莲/旱莲草 (Herba Ecliptae Prostratae) Eclipta	Sweet Sour Cool	KI LR	1. **Nourishes Liver and Kidney Yin:** for dizziness, gray hair, soreness of knees and lower back, insomnia, spermatorrhea, and tinnitus; used with Nu Zhen Zi (as Er Zhi Wan). 2. **Cools Blood and stops bleeding:** for cough with Blood, nose bleeding, Bloody stool, urinary bleeding, and uterine bleeding; used with Che Qian Cao, Bai Mao Gen, Di Yu, E Jiao, Ce Bai Ye.	10-15g
Nu Zhen Zi (Fructus Ligustri Lucidi) 女贞子 Glossy Privet Fruit	Sweet Bitter Neutral	KI LR	1. **Nourishes Liver and Kidney Yin:** for low grade fever, soreness of knee and lower back, dizziness, gray hair, insomnia, spermatorrhea, tinnitus; used with Han Lian Cao. 2. **Blackens hair and brightens eyes:** for poor vision, early gray hair; used with Shu Di Huang, Gou Qi Zi.	10-15g
Hei Zhi Ma	Sweet	KI	1. **Nourishes Liver and**	**10-30g**

(Semen Sesami Idici) 黑芝麻 Black Sesame Seeds	Neutral	LR	**Kidney Yin:** for dizziness, gray hair due to Liver and Kidney essence and Blood Deficiency; used alone or with Shu Di Huang, Zhi Shou Wu, Nu Zhen Zi. 2. **Moistens Intestine:** for constipation due to Blood Deficiency and intestinal Dryness; used with Xing Ren, Bai Shao, Bai Zi Ren.	
Gui Ban (Carapax et Plasttrum Testudinis) 龟板 Tortoise Plastron Fresh Water Turtle Shell	Sweet Salty Cold	HT KI LR	1. **Nourishes Yin and subdues Yang:** for (1) Deficiency Heat, steaming bone symptoms, night sweating due to Yin Deficiency; (2) dizziness due to Yin Deficiency and Yang rising; or (3) tremor of limbs due to Yin Deficiency. A. Internal Wind, used with Sheng Di, Bei Jia, e Jiao (as Da Ding Feng Zhu). B. Hyperactive Liver Yang, used with Niu Xi, Long Gu, Bai Shao, Xuan Shen. 2. **Tonifies Kidney and strengthens bone:** for weakness of low back and knee; fontanel closing, walking and teeth growing delayed in child; used with Hu Gu, Shu Di, Bai Shao (as Hu Qian Wan). 3. **Nourishes Blood and tonifies Heart:** for palpitation, insomnia, poor	**10-25g** Smashed and put early when decocting it. Contraindicated during pregnancy.

			memory due to Heart Blood Deficiency; used with Yuan Zhi, Long Gu. 4. **Stops uterine bleeding:** for excessive uterus bleeding due to Chong and Ren channels not holding; used with Bai Shao, Huang Bai, Xiang Fu (as Gu Jing Wan).	
Bie Jia (Carapax Amydea Sinensis) 鳖甲 Water Turtle Shell	Sweet Slightly Cold	LR KI	1. **Nourishes Yin and subdues Yang:** for (1) Deficiency Heat, steaming bone symptoms, night sweating due to Yin Deficiency; (2) dizziness due to Yin Deficiency and Yang rising; or (3) febrile diseases damaged Yin. A. Yin Deficiency with Heat signs, used with Di Gu Pi, Qin Jiao (as Qin Jiao Bie Jia San). B. Internal Wind due to Yin Deficiency, used with Mu Li, Gui Ban, Sheng Di, E Jiao. 2. **Softens mass and dissipates nodules:** for masses, accumulation, and malaria with palpable masses; used with San Leng, E Zhu, Qing Pi.	**10-25g** Smashed and put early when decocting it. The unprocessed enriches Yin and subdues Yang; Vinegar fried is good at softening hardness and reducing swelling or nodules. Contraindicated during pregnancy.
Gou Qi Zi (Fructus Lycii) 枸杞子 Wolfberry Fruit	Sweet Neutral	LR LU KI	1. **Nourishes Yin and essence:** for soreness of lower back, spermatorrhea, dizziness and diabetes due to Liver and Kidney Yin Deficiency; used with Shu Di Huang, Bai	10-15g

			Shao. 2. **Brightens eyes:** for blurred vision, cataract due to Liver and Kidney Yin Deficiency. with Ju Hua, Shu Di Huang, Shan Yu Rou, Shan Yao (as Qi Ju Di Huang Wan). 3. **Moistens Lung and stops cough:** for cough due to Lung Yin Deficiency; used with Mai Men Dong, Bei Mu	
Sang Shen (Fructus Mori Albea) 桑椹 Mulberry Fruit-Spike	Sweet Cold	HT KI LR	1. **Nourishes Yin and Blood:** for dizziness, tinnitus, blurred vision, insomnia, early gray hair, joint pain, spermatorrhea due to Yin and Blood Deficiency; used with Nu Zhen Zi, He Shou Wu, Shu Di Huang. 2. **Generates fluid and moistens Intestine:** for diabetes, used with Gou Qi Zi, Tian Hua Fen. For constipation due to large Intestine Dryness; used with He Shou Wu, Dang Gui, Huo Ma Ren, Hei Zhi Ma.	10-15g
Yin Er (Fructicato Tremellae) 银耳 White fungus;tremella	Sweet Bland Neutral	LU ST	1. **Nourishes Lung Yin:** for chronic, dry coughing, hemoptysis due to Lung Yin Deficiency. 2. **Nourishes Stomach Yin and generates fluid:** for thirsty, dry mouth due to Stomach Yin Deficiency or febrile diseases damaged Yin.	3-10g

Practice 30

1. Which of the following herbs should be decocted more 30 minutes?
A. Rou Gui
B. Fu Zi
C. Wu Zhu Yu
D. Ding Xiang

2. Which of the following herbs can stop diarrhea?
A. Xiao Hui Xiang
B. Rou Gui
C. Wu Zhu Yu
D. Ding Xiang

3. Which of the following herbs can subdue rebellious Qi for hiccough and vomiting?
A. Xiao Hui Xiang
B. Rou Gui
C. Ding Xiang
D. Gan Jiang

4. Which of the following herbs can Warm Kidney Yang for impotence with lower back and knee soreness?
A. Hua Jiao
B. Gao Liang Jiang
C. Wu Zhu Yu
D. Ding Xiang

5. Which of the following herbs can warm Middle Jiao, alleviate pain and Kill parasites?
A. Rou Gui
B. Ding Xiang
C. Gan Jiang
D. Hua Jiao

6. Lu Rong is:
A. Pungent, warm.
B. Bitter, warm.
C. Sweet, slight warm.
D. Sweet, salty, warm.

7. The herb with pungent, hot and toxic properties is:

A. Xian Mao
B. Ba Ji Tian
C. Yin Yang Huo
D. Bu Gu Zhi

8. The functions of Yin Yang Huo are:
A. Tonify KI Yang, Strengthen bone and sinew and expel Wind-Damp-Cold.
B. Tonify KI and LV, and warm LU.
C. Tonify Yang, transform Cold Phlegm and dry Dampness.
D. Tonify KI and SP, nourish Blood and moisten LU.

9. The herb that treats impotence due to KI Yang Deficiency, and chronic cough with Bloody Phlegm is:
A. Du Zhong
B. Xing Ren
C. Dong Chong Xia Cao
D. Ba Ji Tian

10. The functions of Du Zhong are:
A. Tonify KI and LV, moisten bowel and stop cough.
B. Tonify KI and LV, strengthen the sinews and bones, and calm the fetus.
C. Tonify KI Yang and expel Wind-Damp.
D. Tonify KI and LU, and calm the fetus.

11. The functions of Lu Rong are:
A. Nourish Blood and body essence, and expel Phlegm.
B. Tonify KI Yang, nourish essence, and strengthen the sinews and bones.
C. Tonify LV and KI, moisten bowel and benefit throat.
D. Tonify KI Yang and induce urination.

12. The herb that nourishes LU and ST Yin, and generates body fluid is:
A. Sha Shen
B. Gui Ban
C. Dang Gui
D. Shu Di Huang

13. The functions of Mai Men Dong are:
A. Nourish Yin and moisten LU, generate body fluid to relieve thirst.
B. Nourish LU Yin, nourish ST Yin, and nourish HT Yin.
C. Nourish Yin and moisten LU, tonify SP.
D. Clear Damp-Heat and stop cough

14. The herb that nourishes Yin and suppresses hyperactive Yang, softens the hardness and dissipates nodules is:
A. Nu Zhen Zi
B. Gou Qi Zi
C. Bie Jia
D. Gui Ban

15. The herb that nourishes Yin and tonifies KI, nourishes LV and improves vision is:
A. Nu Zhen Zi
B. Bie Jia
C. Gui Ban
D. Sha Shen

16. Both Gui Ban and Bie Jia can:
A. Nourish LU and ST.
B. Nourish Blood and improve vision.
C. Nourish Yin and suppress hyperactive Liver Yang.
D. Tonify KI and nourish Blood.

17. Both Gui Ban and Bie Jia go to:
A. LU and SP channels.
B. KI and LI channels.
C. KI and LU channels.
D. KI and LV channels.

18. Which of the following herbs treat chronic diarrhea due to Spleen-Kidney Yang Deficiency?
A. Zi Yuan
B. Bu Gu Zhi
C. Rou Cong Rong
D. Du Zhong

19. Which pair of Yang tonifying herb are best to treat low back and knee soreness and weakness due to KI Yang Deficiency?
A. Du Zhong & Tu Si Zi.
B. Du Zhong & Xu Duan.
C. Bu Gu Zi & Xian Mao.
D. Yin Yang Huo & Xian Mao.

20. Which of following Yin tonifying herbs also stops uterine bleeding?
A. Gui Ban
B. Nu Zhen Zi

C. Bai He
D. Sha Shen

21. Both Yu Zhu and Sha Shen:
A. Nourish LV and KI Yin.
B. Clear HT and LU Heat.
C. Stop cough.
D. Nourish LU and ST Yin.

22. Which of the following herbs tonifies LV and KI, promotes mending of the sinews and bones, also stops uterine bleeding and calms the fetus?
A. Shu Di Huang.
B. Sha Shen.
C. Xu Duan.
D. Nu Zhen Zi.

23. The herb that tonifies KI and strengthens Yang, and moistens bowel to relieve constipation is:
A. Rou Cong Rong
B. Shu Di Huang
C. He Shou Wu
D. Dang Gu

Answer Keys: 1B. 2C. 3C. 4D. 5D. 6D. 7A. 8A. 9C. 10B. 11B. 12A. 13B. 14C. 15A. 16C. 17D. 18B. 19B. 20A. 21C. 22C. 23A

Chapter 15 Herbs that Stabilize and Bind

Classification

1. Herbs that stop sweating
2. Herbs that stabilize essence, control urination and excessive vaginal discharge
3. Herbs that astringe Lung and Intestine

Section 1 Herbs that stop sweating

1. Ma Huang Gen (Radix Ephedrae) 麻黄根
2. Fu Xiao Mai (Semen Tritii) 浮小麦
3. Nuo Dao Gen Xu (Radix et Rhizoma Oryzae) 糯稻根须

Name	Property	CN	Main Actions & Indications	Remarks
Ma Huang Gen (Radix Ephedrae) 麻黄根 Ephedra root	Sweet Neutral	LU	**1. Stops sweating:** for spontaneous and night sweating caused by Qi Deficiency, Yin Deficiency; or Qi and Blood Deficiency due to giving birth. A. Spontaneous sweating due to Qi Deficiency, used with Huang Qi, Bai Zhu, Dang Gui. B. Night sweating due to Yin Deficiency, used with Wu Wei Zi, Mu Li C. Postpartum sweating, used with Huang Qi, Dang Gui, Fu Xiao Mai.	3-10g
Fu Xiao Mai (Semen Tritii) 浮小麦 Un-Ripe WHeat Grain	Sweet Salty Cool	HT	**1. Stops sweating:** for spontaneous and night sweating caused by Qi Deficiency. A. Spontaneous sweating due to Qi Deficiency, used with Huang Qi, Mu li B. Night sweating due to Yin	**15-30g** Appendix: **Xiao Mai:** nourishes Heart and

			Deficiency, used with Di Gu Pi, Wu Wei Zi, Huang Bai. **2. Clears Deficiency Heat:** for Deficiency Heat, steaming bone syndrome; used with Gan Cao, Da Zao (as Gan Mai Da Zao Tang).	calms spirit
Nuo Dao Gen Xu (Radix et Rhizoma Oryzae) 糯稻根须 Glutinous Rice root	Sweet Neutral	LV HT	**1. Stops sweating:** for spontaneous and night sweating caused by Lung Qi and Wei Qi Deficiency. A. For spontaneous sweating due to Qi Deficiency, used with Fu Xiao Mai, Ma Huang Gen, Huang Qi B. For night sweating due to Yin Deficiency, used with Mu Li, Fu Xiao Mai, Di Gu Pi. **2. Clears Deficiency Heat:** for Deficiency Heat, steaming bone syndrome; used with Sha Shen, Di Gu Pi.	**15-30g** up to 120g

Section 2 Herbs that Stabilize Essence, Control Urination and Excessive Vaginal Discharge

1. Shan Zhu Yu (Fructus Corni) 山茱萸
2. Lian Zi (Semen Nelumbinis) 莲子
3. Qian Shi (Semen Euryales) 芡实
4. Jin Ying Zi (Fructus Rosae Laevigatae) 金樱子
5. Fu Pen Zi (Fructus Rubi) 覆盆子
6. Hai Piao Xiao (Endoconcha Sepiae) 海螵蛸
7. Sang Piao Xiao (Ootheca Mantidis) 桑螵蛸

Name	Property	CN	Main Actions & Indications	Remarks
Shan Zhu Yu (Fructus Corni)	Sour Slightly	KI LR	**1. Tonifies Kidney and Liver:** for dizziness, lower back and	5-10g 30-60g for

山茱萸 Asiatic Cornelian Cherry Fruit	Warm		knee soreness due to Kidney and Liver Deficiency; used with Shan Yao, Shu Di, Fu Ling, Ze Xie, Mu Dan PI (as Liu Wei Di Huang Wan). **2. Stabilizes essence and controls urination:** for spermatorrhea, frequent urination, and enuresis; used with Jin Ying Zi, Shan Yao, Lu Jiao Jiao. **3. Stops sweating and supports the collapsed:** for excessive sweating due to collapse of Qi and Yang, especially as in shock; used with Long Gu, Mu Li, Fu Zi or Ren Shen. **4. Stabilizes the mense and stops bleeding:** for excessive uterine bleeding due to Kidney and Liver Deficiency; used with Bai Shao, E Jiao.	treating shock. Contraindicated in cases of painful and difficult urination or painful urination due to Damp-Heat.
Lian Zi (Semen Nelumbinis) 莲子 Lotus seed	Sweet Astringent Neutral	HT KI SP	**1. Strengthens Spleen and stops diarrhea:** for chronic diarrhea, poor appetite due to Spleen Deficiency. Usually used with Dang Shen, Fu Ling, and Bai Zhu as in Shen Ling Bai Zhu San. **2. Tonifies Kidney, retains essence:** for spermatorrhea due to Kidney Deficiency. Usually used with Qian Shi, Long Gu as in Jin Suo Gu Jing Wan. **3. Controls urination and**	6-15g Contraindicated in cases with abdominal distention or constipation.

			excessive vaginal discharge: for frequent urination and excessive vaginal discharge due to Spleen and Kidney Deficiency. 4. **Nourishes Heart and calms spirit:** for restlessness, insomnia, palpitation due to Kidney and Heart disharmony; used with Huang Lian, Dang Shen.	
Qian Shi (Semen Euryales) 芡实 Gorgon euryale seed	Sweet Astringent Neutral	KI SP	1. **Strengthenes Spleen and stops diarrhea:** for chronic diarrhea, poor appetite due to Spleen Deficiency; used with Dang Shen, Fu Ling, Bai Zhu. 2. **Tonifies Kidney, keeps essence and control urination:** for spermatorrhea, enuresis due to Kidney Deficiency; used with Jin Ying Zi. 3. **Expels Dampness and controls excessive vaginal discharge:** for excessive vaginal discharge due to Spleen and Kidney Deficiency; used with Shan Yao, Huang Bai, Che Qian Zi.	10-15g
Jin Ying Zi (Fructus Rosae Laevigatae) 金樱子 Cherokee	Sour Astringent Neutral	BL KI LI	1. **Stabilizes essence and controls urination:** for spermatorrhea, frequent urination, enuresis and excessive vaginal discharge;	6-15g Overdose or long-term use may cause abdominal pain

Rosehip			used with Qian Shi, Long Gu, Mu Li. 2. **Strengthens Spleen and stops diarrhea:** for chronic diarrhea, poor appetite due to Spleen Deficiency; used with Dang Shen, Bai Zhu, Shan Yao.	or constipation.
Fu Pen Zi (Fructus Rubi) 覆盆子 Chinese Raspberry	Sweet Astringent Slightly Warm	KI LR	1. **Stabilizes essence and controls urination:** for spermatorrhea, frequent urination, enuresis, and infertility. Usually used with Gou Qi Zi, Tu Si Zi, Wu Wei Zi as in Wu Zi Yan Zong Wan. with Sang Piao Xiao, Yi Zhi Ren. 2. **Improves vision:** for poor vision due to Kidney and Liver Deficiency; used with Du Zhong, Tu Si Zi, Gou Qi Zi.	3-10g 1; used with caution in cases of Yin Deficiency with Heat signs. 2.Contraindicat-ed in cases of urinary difficulty.
Hai Piao Xiao (Endoconcha Sepiae) 海螵蛸 Cuttlefish bone	Salty Astringent Slightly Warm	KI LR ST	1. **Stabilizes essence and controls excessive vaginal discharge:** for spermatorrhea and excessive vaginal discharge; used with Shan Zhu Yu, Tu Si Zi, Sha Yuan Ji Li. 2. **Stops bleeding:** for Stomach bleeding, injury bleeding, and excessive uterine bleeding. 3. **Reduces acidity:** for peptic ulcer; used with Zhe Bei Mu. 4. **Expels Dampness and promote healing:** for chronic eczema, skin ulcer.	6-12g Long term use can cause constipation.

			topically in powdered form	
Sang Piao Xiao (Ootheca Mantidis) 桑螵蛸 Mantis Cradle, Ootheca Mantidis	Sweet Salty Neutral	KI LR	1. **Stabilizes essence and controls urination:** for spermatorrhea, frequent urination, and enuresis; used with Shan Zhu Yu, Qian Shi, Suo Yang. 2. **Tonifies Kidney Yang:** for impotence.	3-10g Contraindicated in cases of Yin Deficiency with Heat signs or Damp-Heat in the bladder.

Section 3 Herbs that Astringe Lung and Intestine

1. Wu Wei Zi (Fructus Schisandrae Chinensis) 五味子
2. Wu Mei (Fructus Mume) 乌梅
3. He Zi (Fructus Chebulae) 诃子
4. Shi Liu Pi (Pericarpium Granati) 石榴皮
5. Wu Bei Zi (Galla Chinensis) 五倍子
6. Rou Dou Kou (Semen Myristicae) 肉豆蔻
7. Bai Guo (Semen Ginkgo) 白果

Name	Property	CN	Actions & Indications	Remarks
Wu Wei Zi (Fructus Schisandrae Chinensis) 五味子 Schisandra Fruit/Seed	Sour Sweet Warm	HT KI LU	1. **Astringes Lung and stops cough:** for chronic cough and wheezing due to Lung and Kidney Deficiency; used with Shu Di Huang, Shan Yu Rou, Shan Yao, Fu Ling (such as Du Qi Wan). 2. **Generates fluid:** for sweating with thirst after due to Heat as in Sheng Mai San, diabetes due to Yin Deficiency. 3. **Stops sweating:** for spontaneous and night sweating due to Qi or Yin Deficiency.	**3-6g** Contraindicated in Exterior syndrome or in the early stages of cough or rashes.

			A. Spontaneous sweating, used with Huang Qi, Sheng Di, Tian Hua Fen. B. Night sweating, used with Zhi Mu , Bai Shao, Fu Xiao Mai. C. Sweating accompanied owith thirsty and palpitation, used with Ren Shen, Mai Dong **4. Stabilizes essence:** for spermatorrhea due to Kidney Deficiency. A. Nocturnal emission, spermatorrhea, Vaginal discharge, used with Sang Piao Xiao, Long Gu. B. Daybreak diarrhea, used with Wu Zhu Yu. **5. Stops diarrhea:** for chronic diarrhea due to Spleen and Kidney Deficiency Cold. **6. Calms Shen:** for insomnia, palpitation, dream disturbed sleep due to Yin and Blood Deficiency or Heart and Kidney Deficiency; used with Suan Zao Ren, Sheng Di Huang.	
Wu Mei (Fructus Mume) 乌梅 Mume	Sour Warm	LI LR LU SP	**1. Astringes Lung and stops cough:** for chronic dry cough due to Lung and Kidney drficiency; used with Ying Su Ke, Ban Xia, Xing Ren, E Jiao. **2. Stops diarrhea:** for chronic diarrhea and dysentery; used with Rou Dou Kou, Dang Shen, He Zi (as Gu Chang Wan). **3. Generates fluid and stops thirst:** for diabetes due to Yin	3-10g

			Deficiency; used with Tian Hua Fen, Mai Men Dong, Ren Shen, (as Yu Quan Wan). 4. **Expels roundworm:** for abdominal pain, vomiting due to roundworm. It is one of the important herbs for treating roundworm; used with Xi Xin, Chuan Jiao, Rou Gui, Fu Zi (as Wu Mei Wan).	
He Zi (Fructus Chebulae) 诃子 Medicine Terminalia Fruit, Fruit of medicine Terminalia	Bitter Sour Astringent Neutral	LU ST LI	1. **Stops diarrhea:** for chronic diarrhea, prolapse of anus due to Deficiency. A. Chronic diarrhea or dysentery from Deficiency Cold, used with Bai Zhu, Rou Dong Kou, Rou Gui, Mu Xiang, Dang Gui (as Zhen Ren Yang Zhang Tang). B. Chronic dysentery with Heat, used with Huang Lian, Mu Xiang, Gan Cao (as He Zi San). 2. **Astringes Lung and stops cough:** for chronic cough, loss of voice due to Lung and Kidney Deficiency. A. Chronic cough, used with Dang Shen, Mai Dong, Wu Wei Zi. B. Hoarseness or loss of voice, used with Jie Geng, Gan Cao (as He Zi Tang).	3-10g 1. Contraindicted for Exterior syndrome 2. Contraindicted for internal accumulation and stagnation of Damp-Heat.
Shi Liu Pi (Pericarpium Granati) 石榴皮	Sour Warm **Toxic**	KI LI ST	1. **Stops diarrhea:** for chronic diarrhea due to Deficiency. 2. **Kills parasites:** for roundworm, tapeworm, and	3-10g It can reduce conceive rate.

Pomegranat e peel			hookworm. **3. Stops bleeding:** for heavy bleeding during menstruation, Blood in the stool.	
Wu Bei Zi (Galla Chinensis) 五倍子 Gallnut of Chinese Sumac	Sour Salty Cold	KI LI LU	**1. Astringes Lung and clears Fire:** for chronic cough due to Lung Deficiency or Lung Heat. **2. Stops diarrhea:** for chronic diarrhea. **3. Stabilizes essence:** for spermatorrhea. **4. Stops sweating:** for spontaneous and night sweating caused by Qi or Yin Deficiency. **5. Stops bleeding:** for Blood in the stool, urine bleeding, and excessive uterine bleeding. **6. Reduces swelling.**	3-9g
Rou Dou Kou (Semen Myristicae) 肉豆蔻 Nutmeg Seeds	Acrid Warm	LI SP ST	**1. Astringes Intestine and stops diarrhea:** for chronic diarrhea due to Spleen and Kidney Yang Deficiency; used with Wu Zhu Yu, Wu Wei Zi, Bu Gu Zhi (as Si Shen Wan). **2. Warms the middle and stops pain:** for Stomach ache, poor appetite and vomiting.	3-10g
Bai Guo (Semen Ginkgo) 白果 Ginkgo Nut	Sweeet Bitter Astringent Neutral **Toxic**	KI LU	**1. Astringes Lung and stops wheezing:** for coughing and wheezing due to Wind Cold, Phlegm, Lung Heat, or Lung Deficiency; used with Ma Huang, Xin Ren, Huang Qi (as Ding Chuan Tang). **2. Stops excessive vaginal discharge:** for excessive vaginal discharge due to	5-10g 1. Contraindicat-ed in cases of excess. 2. Caution whenever there is viscous sputum that is difficult to expectorate.

			Dampness or Spleen and Kidney Deficiency; used with Huang Bai, Qian Shi or Lian Zi, Sang Piao Xiao, Yi Zhi Ren. 3. **Stabilizes essence and control urination:** for spermatorrhea, frequent urination, and enuresis; used with Sang Piao Xiao, Yi Zhi Ren.	3. Should not be taken in large doses or long-term. Overdose leads to headache, fever, tremors, irritability and dyspnea.

Practice 31

1. Astringing herbs have side effect of:
A. Damaging body fluid.
B. Accumulating internal Heat.
C. Retaining pathogens.
D. Dizziness and headache.

2. Which of the following herbs arrests perspiration and calm the spirit?
A. Ren Shen
B. Mai Men Dong
C. Wu Wei Zi
D. Wu Mei

3. The functions of Shan Zhu Yu (Shan Yu Rou) are:
A. Tonify KI and Yang, expel Wind-Damp-Cold.
B. Tonify KI and LV, arrest body essence and sweating, stop bleeding and reduce excessive urination.
C. Tonify Yang, nourish HT and dry Dampness.
D. Tonify KI and SP, nourish Blood and moisten LU.

4. Which of the following herbs does NOT arrest perspiration?
A. Wu Wei Zi
B. Lian Zi
C. Fu Xiao Mei
D. Ma Huang Gen

5. Which of the following herbs tonifies SP and stops diarrhea?
A. Wu Wei Zi
B. Huang Lian
C. Lian Zi
D. Ma Huang Gen

6. The functions of Fu Xiao Mai are:
A. Arrest excessive sweating, and clear Deficiency Heat.
B. Tonify KI Yang, arrest excessive sweating.
C. Tonify LV and KI, moisten bowel and benefit throat.
D. Arrest excessive sweating and diarrhea.

7. The herb that generates body fluid and stop thirst is:
A. He Zi
B. Wu Wei Zi
C. Wu Bai Zi
D. Wu Mei

8. Wu Wei Zi treats chronic cough due to:
A. Dryness in the LU.
B. LU Heat.
C. LU Qi Deficiency.
D. Coldness in the LU.

9. Which of following herbs does NOT stop chronic diarrhea?
A. Wu Wei Zi
B. Wu Mei
C. Rou Dou Kou
D. Ma Hang Gen

Answer Keys: 1C. 2C. 3B. 4B. 5C. 6A. 7D. 8C. 9D

Chapter 16 Herbs that Open the Orifice

Common characters:

1. They are used for treating the closed/locked up disorder (Bi zheng), not abandoned disorder (Tuo zheng).
2. All of them go to Heart channel and most of them are acrid and aromatic.
3. Only use them in lower dosage, short period and taken in pill or powder form.
4. Most of them are contraindicated during pregnancy or Qi, Yin and Blood Deficiency.

Herbs:

1. She Xiang (Secretio Moschus) 麝香
2. Bing Pian (Borneol) 冰片
3. Su He Xiang (Styrax Liquidis) 苏合香
4. Shi Chang Pu(Rhizoma Acori Graminei) 石菖蒲
5. An Xi Xiang (Benzoinum) 安息香
6. Chan Su (Secretio Bufonis) 蟾酥

Name	Property	CN	Actions & Indications	Remarks
She Xiang (Secretio Moschus) 麝香 Navel Gland Secretions of Musk Deer	Acrid Warm Aromatic	**HT** SP LR	**1. Opens orifice and restores Shen:** for coma due to any reason. A. Heat syndrome, with Xi Jiao, Niu Huang (as Zhi Bao Dan) B. Cold syndrome, with Su He Xiang, Ding Xiang (as Su He Xiang Wan). **2. Alleviates pain:** for carbuncle pain and sore throat; used with Mu Xiang, Tao Ren or Su Mu, Mo Yao. **3. Moves Blood:** for amenorrhea, acute chest pain and abdominal pain, masses, injury, Bi syndrome; used with Chi Shao, Dan Shen, San	**0.03-0.1g as powder**. Do not decoct it! 1. Contraindicated during pregnancy. 2; used with caution in cases of hypertension.

			Leng, E Zhu. 4. **Quickens deLivery:** for dystocia, dead fetus or placenta fails to descend; used with Rou Gui, San Leng, E Zhu.	
Bing Pian (Borneol) 冰片 Borneolum syntheticum	Acrid Bitter Cool	**HT** LU SP	1. **Opens orifice and restores Shen:** for coma due to any reason**; used** with She Xiang (as An Gong Niu Huang Wan and Zhi Bao Dan). 2. **Clears Heat and stops pain:** for red eyes, sore throat, mouth sore, otitis media, carbuncles and burn; used with Peng Sha, Mang Xiao, Zhu Sha (as Bing Peng San).	**0.15-0.3g** Do not decoct it! 1. ontraindicated in cases of Qi or Blood Deficiency 2. Caution during pregnancy 3. Do not expose to Heat
Su He Xiang (Styrax Liquidis) 苏合香 Resin of Rose Maloes, Styrax	Sweet Acrid Warm Aromatic	**HT** SP	1. **Opens orifice and restores Shen:** for coma due to Cold or Phlegm; used with Ding Xiang , An Xi Xiang, She Xiang (as Su He Xiang Wan). 2. **Expels filth and stops pain:** for chest and abdominal pain or distention due to Phlegm, Blood stasis or Cold; used with Bing Pian, Tan Xiang.	**0.3-1g** as **powder**. Do not decoct it! 1. Contraindicated in cases of high fever and spontaneous sweating. 2. Caution during pregnancy.
Shi Chang Pu (Rhizoma Acori Graminei) 石菖蒲 Sweetflag Rhizome	Acrid Slightly Warm Aromatic	**HT** ST	1. **Opens orifice and restores Shen:** for coma due to turbid Phlegm, for epilepsy, dizziness, poor memory, tinnitus, deafness due to Phlegm Dampness. A. Deafness, dizziness, forgetfulness, and fulled sensorium, used with Yu Jin, Ban Xia.	3-10g

			2. **Harmonizes Middle Jiao:** for abdominal distention, and dysentery due to turbid Dampness; used with Huo Xiang, Hou Po, Chen Pi.	
An Xi Xiang (Benzoinum) 安息香 Benzoin	Acrid Bitter Neutral	**HT** LR SP	1. **Opens orifice and restores spirit (Shen):** for coma due to any reason. 2. **Moves Blood and stops pain:** for chest and abdominal pain due to Qi and Blood stasis.	**0.6-1.5g** Do not decoct it!
Chan Su (Secretio Bufonis) 蟾酥 Toad Venom, Dried Toad Skin Secretions	Sweet Acrid Warm **Toxic**	**KI** **ST**	1. **Opens orifice and revives Shen (Internally taken):** for coma after vomiting and diarrhea. 2. **Relieves toxicity, reduces swelling and stops pain (Externally use):** for carbuncle, sore throat.	**0.015-0.03g** External use with proper dosage.

Practice 32

1. Besides opening orifices and reviving the spirit, Bing Pian also:
A. Clears Heat and drains Dampness.
B. Clears Heat and generates fluid.
C. Clear Heat and stops pain.
D. Drains Fire and cools Blood.

2. Which of the following herbs clears Heat and opens orifices, clears Liver and extinguishes Wind, and drains Heat and clears Fire toxins?
A. Zhi Zi
B. Nui Huang
C. Shi Chang Pu
D. Huang Lian

3. The functions of Shi Chang Pu are:
A. Open orifices and clear Heat.
B. Open orifices and invigorate Blood.
C. Open orifices and transform Phlegm, harmonize the Middle Jiao and transform Dampness.
D. Clear Damp-Heat and stop bleeding

Answer Keys: 1C. 2A. 3C

Chapter 17 Herbs that Extinguish Wind and Stop Tremor

Common characters:

1. Most of them are animal products.
2. All of them go to Liver channel.
3. Most of them are contraindicated with pregnancy.

Classification:

1. Herbs that extinguish Wind and control spasm and convulsion
2. Herbs that calm Liver and subdue Yang

Section 1 Herbs that Extinguish Wind and Convulsion

1. Ling Yang Jiao (Cornu Saigae Antelopis) 羚羊角
2. Niu Huang (Calculus Bovis) 牛黄
3. Tian Ma(Rhizoma Gaastrodiae Elatae) 天麻
4. Gou Teng (Ramulus cum Uncis Uncariae) 钩藤
5. Di Long (Lumbricus) 地龙
6. Quan Xie(Buthus martensii Karsch) 全蝎
7. Wu Gong (Scolopendra Subspinipes) 蜈蚣
8. (Bai) Jiang Can(Bombyx Batryticatus) 僵蚕

Name	Property	CN	Actions & Indications	Remarks
Ling Yang Jiao (Cornu Saigae Antelopis) 羚羊角 Antelope Horn	Salty Cold	HT **LR**	1. **Extinguishes Liver Wind and stops convulsion:** for (1) spasm and convulsion in febrile diseases and (2) epilepsy due to Liver Wind; used with Gou Teng, Ju Hua, Sheng Di (as Ling Yang Gou Teng Tang). 2. **Subdues Liver Yang:** for dizziness and vertigo due to Liver Yang rising; used with Ju Hua, Shi Jue Ming.	**1-3g** for decoction. Decoct it alone for more than 2 hours. 0.3-0.6g as powder.

			3. **Clears Liver Fire:** for headache, red and swollen eyes, photophobia and lacrimation due to Liver Fire; used with Jue Ming Zi, Huang Qin. 4. **Resolves Fire toxicity:** for high fever with delirium and mania or high fever with erythema and purpura; used with Xi Jiao, Shi Gao. 5. **Stops cough:** for cough and wheezing due to Lung Fire.	
Niu Huang (Calculus Bovis) 牛黄 Cow Gallstone, Ox Gallstone	Bitter Cool	HT **LR**	1. **Extinguishes Liver Wind and stops convulsion:** for spasm and convulsion in febrile diseases due to Liver Wind; used with Gou Teng, Zhu Sha. 2. **Dissolves Phlegm and opens orifices:** for coma, closed mouth; used with She Xiang, Bing Pian (as An Gong Niu Huang Wan). 3. **Clears Heat and resolves toxicity:** for throat pain, mouth sore, carbuncle, scrofula; used with Huang Qin, Xiong Huang (as Niu Huang Jie Du Wan).	**0.2-0.5g**. With caution for pregnant women. 1. It should not be used for conditions that are not associated with Heat excess. 2. Contraindi-cated in cases of Spleen or Stomach Deficiency.
Tian Ma (Rhizoma Gaastrodiae Elatae) 天麻 Gastrodia	Sweet Neutral	**LR**	1. **Extinguishes Liver Wind:** for spasm and convulsion whatever that is Cold or hot, deficient or excess. A. Childhood convulsions, used with Ren Shen, Bai Zhu, Jiang Can B. Seizures, used with Quan Xie. C. Tetany and convulsion, used with Tian Nan Xing, Bai Fu Zi, Qiang Huo.	3-10g Large dose may cause lethargy, reduce deep tendon reflexes, loss of appetite.

			2. **Subdues Liver Yang:** for dizziness and vertigo. 3. **Unblocks channles:** for Bi syndrome; used with Sang Ji Sheng, Qiang Huo, Du Huo (as Zhui Feng Tou Gu Wan).	
Gou Teng (Ramulus cum Uncis Uncariae) 钩藤 Uncaria Hook	Sweet Cool	HT **LR**	1. **Extinguishes Liver Wind:** for spasm and convulsion; used with Ling Yang Jiao, Sang Ye, Ju Hua, Xian Di Huang (as Ling Yang Gou Teng Tang). 2. **Subdues Liver Yang:** for dizziness and vertigo; used with Tian Ma, Huang Qin, Zhi Zi (as Tian Ma Gou Teng Yin).	10-15g. Decoct it within 20 minutes.
Di Long (Lumbricus) 地龙 Earthworm	Salty Cold	BL **LR** LU SP	1. **Clears Heat and extinguishes Wind:** for spasm and convulsion with fever; used along or with Gou Teng, Jiang Can. 2. **Unblocks channels:** for (1)Wind stroke; used with Huang Qi, Dan Gui, Hong Hua (as Bu Yang Huan Wu Tang) **(2)** Bi syndrome. A. Hot obstruction, used with Sang Zhi, Ren Dong Teng, Chi Shao. B. Cold obstruction, used with Chuan Wu, Cao Wu, Nan Xing. 3. **Calms wheezing:** for Lung Heat wheezing. Powdered along or with Ma Huang, Xing Ren. 4. **Promotes urination:** for dysuria. use alone or with Che Qian Zi, Mu.	5-15g. 1-2g as powder.
Quan Xie (Buthus martensii Karsch) 全蝎 Scorpion	Salty Acrid Neutral **Toxic**	**LR**	1. **Extinguishes Liver Wind:** for spasm, convulsion and paralysis due to any reason. A. Acute infantile convulsion with Tian Ma, Gou Teng,Lling. Yang Jiao.	**2-5g** or1-1.5g when just tail is used.

			B. Facial paralysis, with Bai Fu Zi, Jiang Can (as Qian Zheng San) C. Tetanus with Tian Nan Xing, Wu Gong. 2. **Resolves toxicity and dissipates nodules:** for toxic sores and scrofula, external use. 3. **Unblocks channels and stops pain:** for Bi syndrome especially for chronic Bi syndrome with deformed joint, any kind of severe and chronic headache; used with Wu Gong, Jiang Can.	
Wu Gong (Scolopendra Subspinipes) 蜈蚣 Centipede	Acrid Warm **Toxic**	**LR**	1. **Extinguishes Liver Wind:** for spasm, convulsion and paralysis due to any reason. with Quan xie, Jiang Can, Gou Teng. 2. **Resolves toxicity and dissipates nodules:** for toxic sores, scrofula and snake bite. A. Scrofula and sores, used with Xiong Huang topical application. B. Gangrene and ulcerations, used with tea. C. Snakebite, used with Huang Lian, Da Huang, Sheng Gan Cao. 3. **Unblocks channels and stops pain:** for hard treated Bi syndrome, any kind of severe and chronic headache; used with Fang Feng, Du Huo, Wei Ling Xian.	**1-3g.** 0.6-1g as powder.
Jiang Can /Bai Jiang Can (Bombyx Batryticatus) 僵蚕	Salty Acrid Neutral	**LR** LU	1. **Extinguishes Liver Wind:** for spasm and convulsion, especially with Phlegm-Heat. A. Chronic childhood convulsion due to Spleen Deficiency, used with Dang Shen, Bai Zhu, Tian Ma.	3-10g. 1-1.5g as powder.

White Mummified silkworm			B. Seizure due to Phlegm, used with Quan Xie, Tian Ma, Dan Xing C. Facial paralysis due to Wind-Phlegm-Heat, used with Quan Xie, Wu Gong (As Qian Zheng San). 2. **Unblocks channels:** for Wind stroke manifested as facial palsy due to Wind attacking channels. 3. **Expels Wind, stop pain and itching:** for headache, red eyes, throat pain, and lacrimation. A. Headache, red eyes, used with Sang Ye, Ju Hua, Jing Jie. B. Painful, red, swollen throat, used with Jie Geng, Gan Cao, Bo He. 4. **Dissipates nodules:** for Phlegm masses and scrofula; used with Xia Ku Cao, Bei Mu.	

Section 2 Herbs that Subdue Liver Yang

1. Shi Jue Ming (Concha Haliotidis) 石决明
2. Zhen Zhu Mu (Concha Margaritifera) 珍珠母
3. Mu Li (Concha Ostreae) 牡蛎
4. (Dai) Zhe Shi (Haematitum) (代)赭石
5. (Bai/Ci) Ji Li(Fructus Tribuli) (白/茨)蒺藜

Name	Property	CN	Actions & Indications	Remarks
Shi Jue Ming (Concha Haliotidis) 石决明 Abalone Shell	Salty Cold	KI **LR**	1. **Subdues Liver Yang:** for dizziness and vertigo due to Liver and Kidney Yin Deficiency or Liver Fire flaring up with being easily angryed; used with Xia Ku Cao, Gou Teng, Ju Hua, Bai Shao, Mu Li.	**15-30g**.

			2. **Clears Liver and brightens eyes:** for red, swollen, painful eyes due to Liver Fire, or night blindness due to Liver Yin and Liver Blood Deficiency. A. Eye redness, swelling and pain from the upward blazing of Liver Fire, used with Ju Hua, Jue Ming Zi B. Superficial visual obstructions from Wind-Heat, used with Mi Meng Hua, Gu Jing Cao. C. Vision impairment from deficient Liver and Blood, used with Shu Di, Shan Yu Rou (as Shi Ju Ming Wan).	
Zhen Zhu Mu (Concha Margaritifera) 珍珠母 Mother of Pearl	Salty Cold	HT **LR**	1. **Subdues Liver Yang:** for dizziness and vertigo. 2. **Clears Liver and brightens eyes:** for red, swollen, painful eyes, blurred vision, and superficial obstruction. 3. **Clams spirit (Shen):** for insomnia.	**15-30g**. Break and decoct 30 minutes earlier.
Mu Li (Concha Ostreae) 牡蛎 Concha Ostreae	Salty Astringent Cool	KI **LR**	1. **Subdues Liver Yang:** for dizziness and vertigo. with Xuan Shen, Dai Zhe Shi, Long Gu, Chuan Lian Zi 2. **Softens hardness and dissipates nodules:** for Phlegm mass, nodules and scrofula; used with Xuan Shen, Xia Ku Cao, Zhe Bei Mu. 3. **Restrains leakage:** for spermatorrhoea, enuresis, night sweating, spontaneous sweating, and excessive vaginal discharge;	**15-30g**. Break and decoct 30 minutes longer than other herbs.

			used with Chi Shi Zhi. **4. Calms spirit (Shen):** for insomnia; used with Long Gu, Bai Shao.	
Dai Zhe Shi / Zhe Shi (Haematitum) (代)赭石 Hermatite	Bitter Cold	HT **LR** PC	**1. Subdues Liver Yang:** for dizziness and vertigo. with Long Gu, Mu Li, Bai Shao (as Zhen Gan Xi Feng Tang). **2. Guides rebellious Stomach Qi downward:** for vomiting and hiccup; used with Xuan Fu Hua, Ban Xia, Sheng Jiang (as Xuan Fu Dai Zhe Tang). **3. Calms wheezing:** for wheezing due to Lung Qi abnormally go upward or Lung and Kidney Deficiency; used with Dang Shen, Shan Zhu Yu. **4. Cools Blood and stops bleeding:** for bleeding due to Blood Heat. With different herbs according to the syndrome.	**10-30g**. Break and decoct 30 minutes earlier. Use with cauyion for pregnant women.
Bai Ji Li /Ci Ji Li (Fructus Tribuli) (白/刺)蒺藜 Caltrop Fruit, Puncture Vine Fruit	Acrid Bitter Warm **Toxic**	**LR** LU	**1. Subdues Liver Yang:** for dizziness and vertigo. **2. Soothes Liver Qi:** for Liver Qi stagnation. **3. Expels Wind and brighten eyes:** for red, swollen, painful eyes. **4. Expels Wind and stops itching:** for skin lesion with itching.	6-15g
Lu Dou Yi 错误！未找到引用源。 (Glycinis Testa) 橹豆衣 Mung bean skin	Sweet Neutral	**LR**	**1. Subdues Liver Yang:** for dizziness and vertigo.	6-15g

Practice 33

1. The herb that calms Liver and suppresses Liver Yang, cools Blood and stops bleeding, and strongly directs rebellious Qi downward as well is:
A. Long Gu
B. Mu Li
C. Bai Zi Ren
D. Dai Zhe Shi

2. Ling Yang Jiao (cornu antelopis) can be substituted by:
A. Shan Yang Jiao (cornu naemorhedis)
B. Zhi Zi
C. Xi Jiao (cornu rhinoceri)
D. Sheng Di Huang

3. The main functions of Gou Teng are:
A. Regulate Qi and sooth Liver, transform Damp and stop vomiting.
B. Cool Blood and clear Heat, dispel Cold and relieve pain.
C. Extinguish Liver Wind, Subdue Liver Yang.
D. Cool Blood and promote Blood flow, relieve Fire toxins and dissipate nodules.

4. Which of the following herbs dispel Liver Wind as well as stop cough?
A. Tian Nan Xing
B. Mu Dan Pi
C. Tian Ma
D. Ling Yang Jiao

5. Which of the following herbs calms Liver and suppresses Yang, clears Liver Heat and improves vision?
A. Shi Gao
B. Shi Jue Ming
C. Zhi Zi
D. Sheng Di Huang

6. Which channels that Ling Yang Jiao enters to?
A. HT, ST.
B. HT, KI.
C. KI, LV.
D. HT, LV.

7. Which channels do Long Gu and Mu Li enter?
A. HT, LV, ST.
B. HT, LV, KI.
C. KI, LV, LU.
D. HT, LV, LI.

8. Ye Jiao Teng nourishes the Heart and calms spirit, and
A. Nourishes Blood
B. Expels Phlegm
C. Unblock channles
D. Warms the Lung

9. Except calming Liver and anchors Yang, Bai Ji Li also:
A. Drains Dampness.
B. Clears Lung Heat
C. Dispels Wind and stops itching.
D. Calms spirit.

Answer Keys: 1D. 2A. 3C. 4D. 5B. 6D. 7B. 8C. 9C

Chapter 18 Herbs that Expel Parasites

Common characteristics:

1. Can be used for killing parasites in human Intestine
2. Some of them are toxic.
3. Most of them go to SP, ST or LI channels.
4. Some of them can also strengthen Spleen and dissolve accumulation.
5. Usually taken before eating, and with purgatives.
6. Be careful for pregnant women and weak patients.

Herbs

1. Shi Jun Zi (Fructus Quisqualis Indicae) 使君子
2. Ku Lian Pi (Cortex Meliae Radicis) 苦楝根皮
3. Bing Lang (Semen Arecae Catechu) 槟榔
4. Nan Gua Zi (Semen Cucurbitae Moschatae) 南瓜子
5. Da Suan (Bulbus Alli Sativi) 大蒜
6. Fei Zi(Semen Torreyae Grandis) 榧子
7. He Shi (Fructus Carpesii) 鹤虱
8. Lei Wan(Sclerotium Omphaliae) 雷丸
9. Wu Yi(Praeparatio Fructus Ulmi) 芜荑
10. Guan Zhong(Rhizome Guanzhong) 贯众
11. He Cao Ya (Gemma Agrimoniae) 鹤草芽

Name	Property	CN	Actions & Indications	Remarks
Shi Jun Zi (Fructus Quisqualis Indicae) 使君子 Rangoon Creeper Fruit	Sweet Warm	SP ST	1. **Kills parasites:** for roundworm and pinworm. It is one of the important herbs for killing parasites, especially for children; used with Bing Lang, Ku Lian Gen Pi. 2. **Dissolves accumulation:** for childhood malnutritional disorder (Gan Ji) manifested as pale face, skinny body with big	Decoction: 10-15g for adult. For pediatric patients, 1-1.5 piece per year old, maximum 20 pieces per day.

			abdomen; used with Dang Shen, Bai Zhu, Ji Nei Jin.	Do not take it with hot tea and hot food which can lead to hiccup and diarrhea.
Ku Lian Pi (Cortex Meliae Radicis) 苦楝皮 Melia root bark	Bitter Cold **Toxic**	LR SP ST	1. **Kills parasites:** for roundworm, pinworm and hookworm; used with Bing Lang, Bai Bu, Wu Mei. 2. **Treats scabies:** Topically applied for scabies, tinea capitis, tinea cruris, eczema, and impetigo. Mixed with vinegar or oil.	6-9g Contraindicated with Liver diseases patients. Should not be taken long time. Also called Ku Lian Gen Pi.
Bing Lang (Semen Arecae Catechu) 槟榔 Betel Nut, Areca Seeds	Acrid bitter Warm	LI ST	1. **Kills parasites:** for roundworm, tapeworm and pinworm. A. Tapeworms, use alone or with Nan Gua Zi, Fei Zi. B. Pinworm, used with Bai Bu. C. Roundworm, hookworm, used with Ku Lian Pi. 2. **Moves Qi and dissolves accumulation:** for childhood malnutritional disorder (Gan Ji); used with Mu Xiang, Da Huang (as Mu Xiang Bing Lang Wan). 3. **Promotes urination:** for edema. A. Beriberi, used with Mu Gua, Wu Zhu Yu, Zi Su (as Ji Ming San). B. Edema, used with Fu Ling Pi, Ze Xie.	6-15g Good at tapeworm. Be careful for pregnant women.
Nan Gua Zi (Semen Cucurbitae Moschatae) 南瓜子	Sweet Neutral	LI ST	1. **Kills parasites:** for roundworm, tapeworm and schistosome. Usually used with Bing Lang (Semen Arecae Catechu 槟榔). Nan Gua Zi can paralyze the	60-120g taken as powder with room temperature water.

Pumpkin Seeds			middle and late sections of worm and Bing Lang can paralyze the head of worm. A. Tapeworms, used with Bing Lang. B. Roundworm, used with Shi Jun Zi, Wu Mei, Ku Lian Pi.	Also benefited postpartum lactation.
Da Suan (Bulbus Alli Sativi) 大蒜 Garlic	Acrid Warm	LI LU SP	1. **Kills parasites:** for pinworm, hookworm and scabies. 2. **Stops diarrhea:** for dysentery. 3. **Relieves toxicity and reduces swelling:** for carbuncles and scabies. 4. Treat Lung tuberculosis and whooping cough.	5-10g
Fei Zi (Semen Torreyae Grandis) 榧子	Sweet Astringent Neutral	LI LU ST	1. **Kills parasites:** for roundworm, pinworm, fasciolopsis and hookworm. A. Tapeworms, used with Bing Lang. B. Hookworms, used with Bai Bu. C. Roundworms, used with Shi Jin Zi D. Pinworm, used with Bian Xu. 2. **Moistens Intestine:** for constipation due to large Intestine Dryness. 3. **Moisten Lung:** for dry cough due to Lung Dryness.	15-30g It can cause uterus tocontract leading to miscarriage.
He Shi (Fructus Carpesii) 鹤虱 Carpesium Fruit	Bitter Acrid Neutral **Slightly Toxic**	LR	1. **Kills parasites:** for roundworm, pinworm and tapeworm.	5-15g. Do not use it for pregnant women because it can cause abortion.

Lei Wan (Sclerotium Omphaliae) 雷丸 Omphalia fruit	Bitter Cold **Slightly Toxic**	LI ST SP	**Kills parasites:** for tapeworm, roundworm, and hookworm.	6-15g Take it as powder. **Effective ingredient in it will be destroyed if decocted at 60 Centigrade degrees.** Good at tapeworm.
Wu Yi (Praeparatio Fructus Ulmi) 芜荑 Stinking Elm, paste from the fruit	Bitter Acrid Warm	ST	1. **Kills parasites:** for roundworm and pinworm. 2. **Dissolves accumulation:** for childhood malnutritional disorder (Gan Ji).	3-10g
Guan Zhong (Rhizome Guanzhong) 贯众 Cyrtomium Rhizome	Bitter Cold **Slightly toxic**	LR SP	1. **Kills parasites:** for roundworm, tapeworm and pinworm. 2. **Resolves toxicity:** for Wind-Heat, Qi or Blood level Heat and Heat toxicity. 3. **Stops bleeding:** for bleeding due to Blood Heat.	5-10g Do not take fatty food which can accelerate absorption of toxic ingredient.
He Cao Ya (Gemma Agrimoniae) 鹤草芽 Agrimony bud	Bitter Astringe-nt cool	LV SI LI	**Kills parasites:** for tapeworm. It is good at tapeworm and has purgative action.	**30-45g** Take it in the morning before meal. **The effective ingredient does not dissolve in water, so it is taken as powder.**

Practice 34

1. Which of the following action is Shi Jun Zi's action?
A. Kill parasites
B. Stop cough
C. Brighten eyes
D. Tonify Yang

2. Which of the following herbs can NOT kill parasites?
A. Ku Lian PI
B. Fei Zi
C. He Shi
D. Ma Huang

3. Which of the following herbs can NOT kill parasites?
A. Lei Wan
B. Wu Yi
C. He Cao Ya
D. Chai Hu

4. Which of the following action is NOT Bing Lang's action?
A. Kill parasites
B. Move Blood
C. Move Qi and dissolve accumulation
D. Promote urination

5. Which of the following action is NOT Guan Zhong's action?
A. Stop bleeding
B. Calm wheezing
C. Kill parasites
D. Resolve toxicity

6. Nan Gua Zi can
A. Stop bleeding
B. Calm wheezing
C. Kill parasites
D. Resolve toxicity

7. Da Shuan can not

A. Kill parasites
B. Stop diarrhea
C. Relieve toxicity
D. Subdue Liver Yang

Answer Keys: 1A. 2D. 3D. 4A. 5C. 6C. 7D

Chapter 19 Emetic herbs

1. Chang Shan (Radix Dichroae Febrifugae) 常山
2. Gua Di (Pedicellus Cucumeris) 瓜蒂
3. Dan Fan (Chalcanthitum) 胆矾
4. Li Lu (Radix et Rhizoma Veratri) 藜芦

Name	Property	CN	Actions & Indications	Remarks
Chang Shan (Radix Dichroae Febrifugae) 常山 Dichroa root	Bitter Acrid Cold **Toxic**	HT LR LU	1. **Induces vomiting to expel Phlegm:** for Phlegm in the chest. 2. **Checks malaria:** for malaria.	5-10g
Gua Di (Pedicellus Cucumeris) 瓜蒂 Melon Pedicle	Bitter, Cold, **Slightly Toxic**	ST	1. **Induces vomiting:** for Phlegm Heat, retained food 2. **Dispels Damp-Heat:** for jaundice.	**2.5-5g**
Dan Fan (Chalcanthitum) 胆矾 Chalcanthite	Sour, Astringent Acrid **Toxic**	LV LU ST	1. **Induces vomiting:** for epilepsy, seizures, ingestion of poisons. 2. **Resolves toxicity and clears Dampness:** for red eyes, mouth sores, swollen gums.	**0.3-0.6g**
Li Lu (Radix et Rhizoma Veratri) 藜芦 Veratrum root	Cold, Acrid Bitter **Toxic**	LV LU ST	1. **Induces vomiting:** for seizures, ingestion of poisons. 2. **Kills parasites & stops itching:** for scabies, lice, ringworm.	**0.3-0.9g Incompatible with Ren Shen, Dan Shen, Dang Shen, Sha Shen, Ku Shen, Xi Xin, and Shao Yao.**

Practice 35

1. Which of the following herb can NOT induce vomiting?
A. Chang Shan
B. Gua Di
C. Li Lu
D. Sheng Jiang

2. Which of the following herb can not be used with Ren Shen?
A. Chang Shan
B. Gua Di
C. Li Lu
D. Sheng Jiang

Answer Keys: 1D. 2C

Chapter 20 Herbs that Topically Use

Classification:

1. Herbs that kill parasites and stop itching
2. Herbs that pull out toxicity and regenerates flesh
3. Others

Section 1 Herbs that Kill Parasites and Stop Itching

1. She Chuang Zi (Fructus Cnidii Monnieri) 蛇床子
2. Lu Gan Shi (Smithsonitum) 炉甘石
3. Ming Fan (Alumen) 明矾
4. Xiong Huang (Realgar) 雄黄
5. Liu Huang (Sulphur) 硫黄
6. Tu Jing Pi (Cotex Pseudolaricis) 土荆皮
7. Mu Jin Pi (Cotex Hibisci Syriaci) 木槿皮
8. Feng Fang (Nidus Vespae) 蜂房
9. Zhang Nao (Camphora) 樟脑
10. Peng Sha (Borax) 硼砂

Name	Property	CN	Main Actions & Indications	Remarks
She Chuang Zi (Fructus Cnidii Monnieri) 蛇床子 Cnidium Seeds	Acrid Bitter Warm	KI	1. **Dries Dampness, kills parasites and stop itching (Externally use):** for front Yin itching, eczema, scabies; used with Ku Shen, Bai Bu. 2. **Expels Wind and dries Dampness (Internally taken):** for excessive vaginal discharge due to Cold-Dampness, lower back pain due to Dampness. A. Vaginal discharge due to Damp-Cold, used with Shen Zhu Yu, Xiang Fu, Che Qian Zi.	Internal use: 3-10g. External use: 15-30g Contraindicated in cases of Damp-Heat in the lower-jiao and Yin Deficiency with Heat signs.

			B. Lower back pain due to Wind-Damp-Cold, used with Sang Ji Sheng, Du Zhong, Qin Jiao. 3. **Warms Kidney and Tonifies Yang (Internally taken):** for impotence, infertility. with Tu Si Zi, Wu Wei Zi.	
Lu Gan Shi (Smithsonitum) 炉甘石 Calamine Lotion	Sweet Bitter Cold	LR LI SP	1. **Brightens eyes and removes superficial visual obstruction (Externally use):** for red, swollen eyes, eczema. 2. **Dries Dampness and generates flesh (Externally use):** for skin ulcer.	Only for external use with proper dosage. $ZnCO_3$ is in it.
Ming Fan (Alumen) 明矾 Alunite	Sour Astringent Cold	LI LR LU SP ST	1. **Relieves toxicity, kills parasites and stops itching (Externally use):** for eczema, scabies, mouth ulcer, and carbuncle; used with Ban Mao, Bing Pian. 2. **Stops bleeding (Int. & Ext. use):** for epistaxis, vomiting Blood, Blood in stools, and excessive uterine bleeding. 3. **Stops diarrhea (Internally taken):** for chronic diarrhea and dysentery. 4. **Resolves Phlegm (Internally taken):** for coma, epilepsy and mania due to Phlegm.	**0.6-1.5g** 1. Contraindicated during pregnancy. 2. Contraindicated in cases of Yin Deficiency with Heat signs. 3; used with caution for internal use.
Xiong Huang (Realgar) 雄黄 Realgar	Acrid Bitter Warm **Toxic**	HT LR ST	1. **Relieves toxicity, and stop itching (Externally use):** for carbuncle, boil, insect or snake bite. 2. **Kills parasites (Internally taken):** for roundworm; used with Bing Lang, Qian Niu Zi	External use with proper dosage. **0.05-0.3g if used internally.** It contains As_2O_3. Do not use it long time.

			(as Qian Niu Wan).	
Liu Huang (Sulphur) 硫黄 Sulfur	Sour Hot **Toxic**	KI LI	1. **Relieves toxicity, kills parasites and stops itching (Externally use):** for scabies, tinea, and genital itching. 2. **Tonifies Yang (Internally taken):** for Cold type wheezing, impotence, Cold type constipation.	External use with proper dosage. Internal use 1-3g. Contains sulphur. **Antagonistic with Mang Xiao**
Tu Jing Pi (Cotex Pseudolaricis) 土荆皮 Cortex Pseudolaricis ; Chinese golden larch	Acrid Bitter Warm **Toxic**	KI	1. **Kills parasites and stop itching (Externally use):** for many kinds of tinea.	External use with proper dosage.
Mu Jin Pi (Cotex Hibisci Syriaci) 木槿皮 Hibiscus root Bark	Sweet Neutral	LR ST	1. **Kills parasites and stops itching (Externally use):** for scabies, tinea. 2. **Clears Damp-Heat (Ext. & Int.use):** for excessive vaginal discharge and itching due to Damp-Heat.	3-10g External use with proper dosage.
Feng Fang (Nidus Vespae) 蜂房 Wasp nest	Sweet Neutral **Toxic**	LU ST	1. **Relieves toxicity, kills parasites and stops itching (Externally use):** for carbuncle, scrofula, tinea, and scabies. 2. **Expels Wind and stops pain (Ext. & Int. use):** for Bi syndrome, toothache.	Internal use 6-12g as decoction and **1.5-3g** as powder. External use with proper dosage.
Zhang Nao (Camphora) 樟脑 Camphor	Acrid Hot **Toxic**	HT SP	1. **Expels Wind-Dampness, kills parasites and stops pain (Externally use):** for scabies, skin ulcer, scrofula, toothache, injury.	External use with proper dosage. Internal use **0.1-0.2g** as powder.

			2. **Opens orifice and expels filth (Internally taken):** for vomiting and diarrhea with abdominal pain, coma.	
Peng Sha (Borax) 硼砂 Borax	Sweet Salty Cool	LU ST	1. **Clears Heat and relieves toxicity (Externally use):** for sore throat, mouth ulcer, canker sore, red and swollen eyes; used with Bing Pian, Ming Fan. 2. **Clears Lung Heat and dissolves Phlegm (Internally taken):** for coughing with yellow, sticky Phlegm due to Phlegm-Heat; used with Gua Lou, Zhe Bei Mu.	External use with proper dosage. Internal use **1.5-3g**. 1. Caution when using internally. 2. Long-term use can cause renal dysfunction.

Section 2 Herbs that Pull out Toxicity and Generate Flesh

1. Qing Fen (Calomelas) 轻粉
2. Mi Tuo Seng (Lithargyrum) 密陀僧
3. Qian Dan (MInium) 铅丹

Name	Property	CN	Main Actions & Indications	Remarks
Qing Fen (Calomelas) 轻粉 Calomel, Mercurous Chloride	Acrid Cold **Toxic**	BL KI LR	1. **Pulls out toxicity, generates flesh and kill parasites (External use):** for scabies, syphilis, skin ulcer. 2. **Promotes urination and moves bowels (Internal taken):** for edema and constipation.	External use with proper dosage. Internal use **0.1-0.2g** as powder. Contains Hg_2Cl_2.
Mi Tuo Seng (Lithargyrum) 密陀僧 Litharge	Salty Acrid Neutral **Toxic**	LR SP	1. **Pulls out toxicity, generates flesh, and absorbs fluid (External use):** for skin ulcer, eczema, scabies, underarm odor.	External use with proper dosage. Internal use **0.2-0.5g** as powder.

				Contains PbO. Antagonistic to **Lang Du**
Qian Dan (MInium) 铅丹 Plumbum Rubrum	Acrid Cool **Toxic**	HT LR SP	**1. Pulls out toxicity and generates flesh (Externally use):** for skin ulcer, eczema. **2. Checks malaria (Internally taken):** for malaria.	External use with proper dosage. Internal use **0.3-0.6g** as powder. Main ingredient is Pb_3O_4.

Practice 36

1. Liu Huang can not be used with
A. Mang Xiao
B. Da Hung
C. Fan Xie Ye
D. Can Cao

2. Ming Fan can NOT
A. Stop bleeding
B. Kill parasites and stop itching
C. Stop diarrhea
D. Nourish Yin

3. Besides relieve toxicity, and stop itching (External use), Xiong Huang can also
A. Kill parasites (Internally taken)
B. Stop cough
C. Brighten eyes
D. Tonify Yang (Internal use)

4. Besides Relieve toxicity, kill parasites and stop itching (Externally use), Liu Huang also
A. Stop cough
B. Brighten eyes
C. Tonify Yang (Internal taken)
D. Dry Dampness and generate flesh

5. Peng Sha can
A. Stop diarrhea
B. Tonify Yang
C. Nourish Yin
D. Clear Heat and relieve toxicity

6. Lu Gan Shi can Not
A. Stop cough
B. Brighten eyes
C. Remove superficial visual obstruction
D. Dry Dampness and generate flesh

7. Lu Gan Shi is used

A. Topically
B. Orally
C. Both of the above
D. Non of the above

8. Which of the following topically used herb is NOT toxic?
A. Peng Sha
B. Liu Huang
C. Xiong Huang
D. She Chuang Zi

9. Which is NOT the action of She Chuang Zi?
A. Kill parasites and stop itching
B. Expel Wind and dry Dampness
C. Warm Kidney and Tonify Yang
D. Stop pain

Answer Keys: 1A. 2D. 3A. 4C. 5D. 6A. 7A. 8D. 9D

Index

